YOUR GENES, YOUR HEALTH AND PERSONALISED MEDICINE

RC Michaelis

Department of Biology
Western Carolina University

KM Sweet

Division of Human Genetics
The Ohio State University

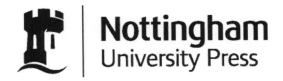

Nottingham
University Press

Nottingham University Press
University of Nottingham, King's Meadow Campus
Lenton Lane, Nottingham, NG7 2NR, England

NOTTINGHAM

First published 2012
© Nottingham University Press

British Library Cataloguing in Publication Data
Your Genes, Your Health And Personalised Medicine

ISBN 978-1-907284-16-8

Disclaimer

Every reasonable effort has been made to ensure that the material in this book is true, correct, complete and appropriate at the time of writing. Nevertheless the publishers and the author do not accept responsibility for any omission or error, or for any injury, damage, loss or financial consequences arising from the use of the book. Views expressed in the articles are those of the author and not of the Editor or Publisher.

Typeset by Nottingham University Press, Nottingham

Printed and bound by Berforts Group, Hertfordshire, England

DEDICATIONS

I dedicate this book to all my students at Western Carolina University. A wise man once told me if you have a job you truly love, you'll never work a day in your life. I am happy to say I am living proof of this. Thank you all.

Ron Michaelis

I dedicate this book to the many people who have touched my life with their own stories, and inspired me to write.

Kevin Sweet

CONTENTS

Contents

5   USING GENETIC TESTING TO MAINTAIN YOUR HEALTH AND PERSONALISE YOUR MEDICAL CARE, NOW AND IN THE FUTURE   89

6   MAKING THE DECISION WHETHER OR NOT TO HAVE GENETIC TESTING, AND INTERPRETING THE RESULTS OF TESTS YOU CHOOSE TO HAVE PERFORMED   109

INTRODUCTION

Personalised Medicine Recognises That You Are A Unique Individual

Improving The Disease-Oriented Approach To Medicine

There is no need to tell you that you are a unique individual. You already know that nobody else has your particular combination of height, weight, skin tone, hair color, personality, sense of humor, skill at sports and games, and love of your favorite food. It isn't just the characteristics you can see about a person that vary from person to person, however. Many aspects of our biology, including processes that help maintain our health, are also highly variable between individuals.

Unfortunately, our medical system often does not treat you as a unique individual. Our medical system often takes a disease-oriented approach to your health; anyone who has a particular disease is treated the same way. If you get sick, and there are several choices of drug and dose your doctor can prescribe, he/she often has no way of knowing which drug and dose will be safest and most effective for you. Your doctor often must follow a trial-and-error strategy to determine the best drug and dose to prescribe.

One of the other important drawbacks to our disease-oriented medical system is the fact that the system places much more emphasis on treating people after they get sick than it does on helping people keep from getting sick. Many people are interested in understanding how to prevent disease, and to stay as healthy as possible as they grow older.

Personalised Medicine Sees You As An Informed, Empowered And Active Participant

One of the goals of personalised medicine is to provide doctors with the information they need in order to prescribe the safest and most effective treatments for you. Some of the personalised medicine tests that are being developed are intended to tell the doctor which of several drugs is most likely to benefit you most, and whether you should get the same dose most people need, or whether you would be better off with a lower or higher dose than that. Personalised medicine doesn't just restrict itself to helping your doctor play his/her role in your health care more effectively, however; it will also allow you to play a more active role in maintaining your own health than you may be accustomed to playing. As we discuss in Chapter 4, one of the keys to this is knowing more about your family's medical history, and understanding how that information can be used to estimate your risk for specific diseases.

One very useful thing that personalised medicine tests will do is inform people about their level of risk for specific diseases. This is done by analysing that person's family history, and when appropriate, by performing specific gene tests. Knowing the diseases for which you have the greatest genetic risk may help you identify ways in which you can adjust your diet, environment or lifestyle (*e.g.* the nongenetic factors) to reduce your overall risk of developing those diseases.

Our current system of medicine does not place much emphasis on the fact that we can all do things to improve our health and reduce our chances of developing specific diseases. Personalised medicine encourages all of us to take a more active role in maintaining our health. In fact, some authorities use the (copyrighted) term **P4 Medicine**™ to symbolise the new approach to health and health care. The term P4 stands for "Predictive, Preventive, Personalised and Participatory." One of the ideas personalised medicine was founded upon is the idea that, if you inform people about the diseases for which they have the highest risk (personal and predictive), they can adopt habits regarding their diet, environment and lifestyle (participatory) that can reduce their risk of developing the disease (preventive). The more we can inform people about the genetic and nongenetic factors that influence their risk for diseases, the more effective they can be at maintaining their own health.

This Book Is Intended To Help You Understand These Important Principles

One of the goals of this book is to help you understand the way in which our family history, our genes, our proteins (which are made by our genes) and things we encounter from our diet, environment and lifestyle interact to influence your risk for diseases or response to a drug. The vast majority of diseases that most people suffer from, and the diseases you are most likely to develop as you grow older, are multifactorial diseases. As the name implies, there are many different genetic and nongenetic factors that can cause a multifactorial disease. In most cases, multifactorial diseases are caused by an interaction between genetic factors the person was born with and nongenetic factors the person encountered through his/her diet, environment and lifestyle over the course of his/her lifetime.

The earliest studies in the field of personalised medicine were focused on understanding the means by which our genes make our proteins, and how the activities of our genes and proteins are regulated. More recently, however, researchers have come to discover that our genes do not control our development, our traits or our health by themselves. Our genes play their role by making our proteins, which perform many of the functions that are required to keep us healthy. Our proteins, however, interact with other proteins, hormones, the things we eat and drink, and agents from our environment such as smoke or the sun's ultraviolet (UV) rays. Our genes are also acted upon directly by the things we encounter through our diet, environment and lifestyle. This complex interplay begins even before you are conceived; recent studies suggest that nongenetic factors that influence the activity of your parents' genes can influence the activity of your genes and proteins. One goal of this book is to help you better understand what the genetic and nongenetic factors are that influence your risk of developing diseases, and appreciate how complex their interactions are.

Another goal of this book is to help you understand how you can use the family history information that you already have available to you to better estimate your level of risk for the diseases that have affected your family members. Most people understand that their family history contains important information, but few know how to properly interpret their family history to accurately estimate their level of risk for the diseases that have appeared in their family members.

A thorough family history not only provides information that helps you estimate your level of genetic risk for the diseases that have affected your family members, but it may also identify the nongenetic factors that contributed to their diseases as well. Having both types of information in your family history may help you estimate your risk of developing the diseases that have affected your family members, as well as identify adjustments you can make in your diet, environment and lifestyle to reduce your overall risk of developing those diseases. There are several Internet websites that contain programs that can help you collect and interpret your family history. These programs are free and accessible to the public, and allow you to produce a summary that you and your doctor can analyse to interpret the significance of your family medical history as effectively as possible.

Understanding the information in this book will allow you to play a more active role in maintaining your own health. In addition, it will allow you to be a better-informed consumer of the genetic testing and personalised medicine services that are available now, and those that will emerge over the next few decades. Some of these companies will advertise some of their services directly to consumers. All their advertisements and information brochures will emphasise the potential benefits that their services may provide you. Understanding the material in this book will enable you to understand what the limitations of these tests are, and decide for yourself whether these new tests will provide truly useful information for you or not.

Personalised Medicine Tests Can Help In Many Ways Throughout Your life

Whole-genome sequencing (WGS) will ultimately be the cornerstone of the genetic tests that are included in personalised medicine tests. Whole-genome sequencing is a procedure that produces the entire sequence of a person's DNA, and thereby provides information about every genetic risk factor the person possesses. A WGS analysis will identify millions of sequence variations in the typical person. Some of these sequence variations will increase the person's risk of developing some of the common adult diseases such as cardiovascular disease, diabetes and various cancers. Others may increase his/her risk of developing psychiatric diseases. Because of the tremendous amount of information that is obtained from a WGS analysis, these tests will impact the typical person's health care in a number of ways throughout his/her life. For example, imagine the following scenario, set in the year 2022:

> Emily, age 23 years, visits with her primary care doctor and asks to have a WGS analysis performed to determine the entire sequence of her DNA. Many of her friends have had their DNA sequenced, and have been discussing the results of their tests through their favorite interactive social media. Emily is primarily concerned about her genetic risks for type 2 diabetes and colon cancer. Both her mother and maternal aunt (her mother's sister) have type 2 diabetes. In addition, her paternal uncle (her father's brother) died of colon cancer when he was 62.

> Emily's doctor agrees that having Emily's DNA sequenced will provide a lot of information, not only about her risks for type 2 diabetes and colon cancer, but also about her risks for other diseases, her physical traits and her ancestry as well. Emily and her doctor also discuss the fact that your genes do not determine your health single-handedly, and that nongenetic factors, including many that you can control, also play an important role in maintaining your health. The doctor contacts a genetic counselor and they work together with Emily. They discuss Emily's personal and family history, review several possible results that the tests might produce, and prepare Emily to cope with the potential psychological impact of the test results.

> The sequencing test reveals that Emily has genetic factors that slightly increase her risk for type 2 diabetes above the typical person's risk, and other genetic factors that significantly increase her risk for colon cancer above the typical person's risk. Emily also has genetic factors that reduce her risk for asthma and Alzheimer disease.

Emily also carries a number of gene mutations that could factor into her children's health if she should choose to have children some day. For example, Emily is found to carry a gene mutation that causes a very severe childhood disease, spinal muscular atrophy (SMA). This mutation is a recessive mutation (discussed in Chapter 3), however. This means that the person will not develop the disease unless he/she has the mutation in both of his/her two copies of the corresponding gene. Because Emily only has the mutation in one copy of the gene, Emily does not have SMA. If Emily decides to have a child some day, however, she has a 50% chance of passing the mutation down to the child. If Emily's partner also carries a recessive mutation in the same gene, and both parents pass the mutation down to the child, the child will be affected with SMA. This information is significant not only for Emily, but also for several of her family members, who may also possess this recessive mutation.

Because controlling your weight reduces your risk for type 2 diabetes, Emily's doctor brings a nutritionist into the discussion, and together they recommend that Emily make a few changes in her diet, begin a program of exercise and get her blood sugar level monitored regularly. These modifications in her diet and lifestyle greatly reduce the chance that Emily will develop type 2 diabetes.

Because she has an elevated genetic risk for colon cancer, Emily is advised to make a few changes in her diet, such as reducing her consumption of barbecued meat, and increasing her intake of soy-based foods and fiber. This recommendation is based not only on an analysis of Emily's genetic sequence, but also on a test that has determined the particular types of bacteria Emily has in her digestive system.

Although dietary adjustments such as these may reduce some people's risk of developing colon cancer, Emily's genetic factors have increased her risk for colon cancer to a high enough level that dietary manipulations may not be able to prevent her from developing colon cancer. Emily therefore begins undergoing colorectal screening tests at age 25, rather than at 50, when most people begin this procedure, and has the screenings more frequently than is recommended for most other people. At age 45, a pre-cancerous polyp is detected and successfully removed. Another pre-cancerous polyp is detected and removed when Emily is 52, and another when she is 65. Despite the fact that several pre-cancerous polyps develop over the course of her lifetime, Emily never develops colon cancer.

When she turns 30, Emily gets married and would like to have children. Because Emily carries several recessive mutations that can seriously impair her children's health, her husband Conner wants to be tested to see if he also carries recessive mutations in the same genes. Together, they contact a genetic counselor and Conner's medical and family history is explored. Conner undergoes WGS, and although he is found to have a number of genetic risk factors for common diseases (as was seen with Emily), including several recessive mutations that could cause serious diseases in his children if they inherited the mutation from both parents, he does not have any mutations in the same genes in which Emily has her recessive mutations.

Fifteen years later, Emily develops mild asthma. The fact that DNA sequencing did not reveal any genetic factors that increased Emily's risk for asthma illustrates the importance of nongenetic factors in influencing a person's risk for many diseases. Emily has been using monitors that show that she is exposed to second-hand smoke and other allergens. In addition, she sometimes jogs in cold weather. Her healthcare team advises her that both these environmental factors can contribute to asthma. They recommend that she jog indoors in the winter, and they work with Emily to develop a plan that reduces her exposure to these environmental factors.

In spite of the fact that genetic testing did not predict that Emily would develop asthma, it can still help Emily's doctor treat her in the safest and most effective manner possible. Emily's doctor has a number of drugs he/she commonly prescribes for patients with asthma. Her WGS analysis shows that Emily has a genetic factor that is associated with a good response to one of the drugs in particular, and Emily's doctor prescribes that drug as a first line treatment. In addition, the WGS also revealed that Emily is a slow metaboliser of that drug, and therefore needs to be given a lower dose than the average person starts with. The medication helps relieve Emily's asthma symptoms, and she experiences no adverse side effects.

Emily's story illustrates only a few of the ways in which personalised medicine tests will impact your ability to maintain your own health and your health care providers' abilities to provide you the safest and most effective treatments. As the field of personalised progresses, personalised medicine tests will go beyond genetic tests. Personalised medicine tests will eventually combine genetic information with information about your blood chemistry (proteins, sugar, fats), current medical condition (blood pressure, weight), family medical history and personal characteristics such as age and sex. These tests will enable you and your doctor to estimate your risk for specific diseases more accurately. Knowing which diseases you have the greatest risk for may enable you to play a more active role in maintaining your own health, by reducing your exposure to some of the nongenetic factors that increase your risk of developing that disease.

Emily's story also illustrates how important it will be to counsel people regarding the potential psychological impact of genetic testing. Helping the person prepare for the possible psychological impact of genetic testing is important now, but will become especially important once WGS becomes routine. A WGS analysis will identify millions of sequence variations in the typical person. Some of these sequence variations will increase the person's risk of developing some of the common adult diseases such as cardiovascular disease, diabetes and various cancers. Others may increase his/her risk of developing psychiatric diseases or other behavioral traits. If these diseases have not appeared in that person's family yet, this surprising news may add to whatever anxiety the person may have already been feeling about his/her risk for the diseases that have affected his/her family members. Because the results of genetic (and other) tests can have such a profound psychological impact on the person, it will always be essential to provide proper counseling, to maximise the benefits of personalised medicine testing and reduce the chances that the information will cause someone undue distress.

In addition, there will always be situations in which the genetic counselor must help the person cope with a situation over which he/she has no control. Researchers are continually learning more about the nongenetic factors that influence your risk for disease, and as the field of personalised medicine progresses there will be many situations in which the person can adjust his/her diet, environment or lifestyle to reduce his/her overall risk of developing the disease. There will always be some situations, however, in which the person will not be able to influence his/her risk for the disease by adjusting his/her diet, environment and lifestyle; these may be especially anxiety-provoking.

THE FIELD OF PERSONALISED MEDICINE IS STILL DEVELOPING, BUT ALL THE ELEMENTS ARE COMING TOGETHER

In time, the field of personalised medicine will develop to a point at which Emily's story will be a model for the average person's health care. Two of the biggest obstacles to progress in this field are the cost of DNA sequencing technology and the challenge of being able to interpret the huge amount of information that is produced when you determine a person's entire DNA sequence. This latter challenge is a significant one. Different genetic and nongenetic factors interact in a variety of different ways, and the significance of some genetic and nongenetic factors changes as you get older. Gathering the DNA sequence information is relatively easy. Figuring out exactly which genetic and nongenetic factors to consider, and whether to consider some factors more influential than others, is the true challenge facing researchers who are trying to develop personalised medicine tests.

Both these problems are being overcome by new technologies. New sequencing technologies are being developed that will bring the cost of sequencing down significantly in the near future. In addition, a number of other tests are being developed that focus on proteins, fats, sugars and other important aspects of your personal biochemistry. New computer technologies are also being developed that will enable analysts to make the most out of the information that DNA sequencing provides. As researchers identify more of the genetic and nongenetic factors that influence our risk for diseases, these new computer programs will better enable them to determine exactly how to combine the different factors into a formula that predicts your risk for a disease as accurately as possible. In addition, as we learn more about the nongenetic factors that influence our risks for diseases, there will be more situations in which your health care team can make recommendations for diet, environment and lifestyle changes that will reduce your risk of developing the disease in question.

As the cost of sequencing drops, more researchers find themselves able to use sequencing to collect ever-increasing amounts of data from their subjects. The ability to collect and interpret ever-increasing amounts of genetic data has increased the pace of new discoveries, which will increase the pace at which new, and more useful, tests emerge. In addition, as the cost of genetic testing declines, insurance companies may be more inclined to cover the cost of these tests, thereby increasing their use in different areas of medicine.

In the not too distant future, personalised medicine will be the standard of care in every field of medicine. There will also be a lot of genetic tests and other personalised medicine tests that are offered by commercial testing companies that may sound intriguing, but produce little information that is of real use to you or your doctor. We hope this book helps you better understand what these personalised medicine tests are all about, and how to differentiate between those tests that are truly useful and those that are not. Perhaps most importantly, we hope this book helps you identify ways in which you can improve your own health, by controlling the dietary, environmental and lifestyle factors that contribute to the diseases for which you have the greatest risk.

Ron Michaelis
Kevin Sweet

CHAPTER 1

UNDERSTANDING THE MEANS BY WHICH OUR GENES INFLUENCE OUR HEALTH

THE FIELD OF PERSONALISED MEDICINE GOT OFF TO A SLOW START, BUT IT HAS PICKED UP CONSIDERABLE SPEED

It All Started With A Mouse

That may sound like the title to a documentary about Walt Disney, but actually, a mouse with an unusual characteristic did begin the process that has led us to the era of personalised medicine. The idea that we are all individuals in the biochemical sense was first formalised in the scientific literature around 1902, when Archibald Garrod (who was later made Sir Archibald Garrod, in recognition of his important work in biochemistry) coined the term "biochemical individuality." Garrod was doing research using mice as subjects, when he noticed that the bedding in one of his mouse cages turned black after the mice urinated on it.

The black color was due to a substance called homogentisic acid that is not usually present in the urine of mice. There had been a change in the DNA sequence of one of Garrod's mice, which in turn changed the way the mouse's body processed proteins. This resulted in the mouse having homogentisic acid in its urine, which turned black after it sat in the air for a while. One of the most interesting things Garrod observed was that the mice that had this gene mutation did not have any noticeable physical or behavioral abnormalities. Garrod's work demonstrated that there are some individuals in a population whose biochemistry is different from that of the other individuals in the same population, and that these differences do not necessarily cause those individuals to have diseases. We now know that this principle applies not only to mice, but to all living creatures, including people.

By the time Garrod published his work, the science of genetics had already been founded. Gregor Mendel (1822-1884) had presented his pioneering work on the inheritance of traits in pea plants in 1865. While Mendel's theories were generally well-received by the scientific community, they were not given a great deal of publicity; Mendel was a monk, so his traveling and lecturing was limited.

Genetics was drawn into the public spotlight, however, when Charles Darwin (1809-1882) published his theory about evolution (Darwin's book *On The Origin Of Species* was published in 1859). Darwin's theory of evolution was built upon genetic principles, and also emphasised how important individual differences were in determining which individuals thrived better in their environment.

The concept of individual differences, and the ability to pass down our traits to our children, was also the foundation for the work of Francis Galton (1822-1922). Galton (Darwin's half-cousin) published notable works in several fields, including the inheritance of intelligence, in the 1860s-1880s. Galton was so convinced that intelligence was an inherited trait that he offered his daughters large sums of money as incentives to marry and have children with university professors. His work gave rise to movements that encouraged intelligent people to mate with other intelligent people, as well as programs to sterilise mentally handicapped people as a means of reducing the frequency of their "bad" genes in the gene pool.

The process whereby you try to improve the human gene pool by selective mating is called **eugenics**. Galton's work inspired a number of countries to institute eugenics programs. Some programs practice positive eugenics, in which people with desirable characteristics are encouraged to mate. Other programs practice negative eugenics, in which people who have undesirable characteristics are sterilised to prevent them from mating. Many of these programs focused on sterilising people who had mental handicaps. Some people objected to these eugenic programs on ethical grounds, but many American states and several other countries had negative eugenics programs before World War II. It wasn't until Adolf Hitler instituted a negative eugenics program that went well beyond most people's ethical boundaries that negative eugenics programs were terminated. Positive eugenics programs are still active, though. Sperm and egg banks are examples of institutionalised positive eugenics programs. In addition, we all practice positive eugenics on the personal level, merely by selecting people who have characteristics we consider desirable as our mates.

It Took 50 Years For The Field Of Personalised Medicine To Begin Developing

Despite the fact that Garrod's concept of biochemical individuality was well received by the scientific community, and built upon generally-accepted principles of genetics and inheritance, the first application of this concept to medicine didn't appear until the late 1950's, when three studies were published that described how some people responded differently to certain medications than others. These studies reported that some people's bodies metabolise (break down and get rid of) prescription drugs faster than other peoples' bodies do, and that those people who were slow metabolisers were more likely to have dangerous side effects when given those particular drugs than fast metabolisers were. One study showed that more black people were slow metabolisers of a drug called primaquine (which is prescribed for people with malaria or pneumonia) than white people were, thereby explaining why black people were more likely than white people to develop a particular blood disease after being given primaquine. Another reported that different people metabolised the tuberculosis drug isoniazid at different rates, and that tuberculosis patients who were slow metabolisers had a higher than average risk for nerve damage after isoniazid. The third of these pioneering studies reported that people who metabolised certain anesthetics slowly had a higher risk for paralysis of the respiratory system than other people did.

In all three cases, further research revealed that a variation in a gene's sequence caused that gene's protein to have a lower level of activity in some people than in others. Because these particular proteins help your body metabolise these drugs, having the slower-acting version of the protein caused that person to build up a higher concentration of the drug in his/her body, and made him/her more likely to have a dangerous reaction to the drug. These studies all illustrated a principle that is one of the cornerstones of personalised medicine:

> The individual's genetic status interacts with nongenetic factors (in this case, the drug) to determine the state of the individual's health at any given time.

These cases made it clear that people could have unusual genetic features, but not be obviously affected by a disease. The people who had the dangerous reactions to the drugs did not have obvious genetic diseases. The specific variations they possessed of the genes in question did not impair their development in general. In fact, these people could have lived long lives and never known they had that important risk-increasing gene variation, if they had not been prescribed those specific drugs. It wasn't until their genetic predisposition had the opportunity to interact with the critical nongenetic factor (the drug) that their genetic status became apparent.

Throughout the 1970s-1990s, the field of genetics bloomed, primarily because there were a great many advances made in the technology used for DNA analyses. The focus of many of the studies from this era was on gene mutations that were capable of causing a genetic disease all by themselves (these diseases are referred to as **single-gene diseases**, and will be discussed in Chapter 3). These discoveries explained the cause of disease for millions of people. Collectively there are more than 6,000 different single gene disorders, and they affect approximately 4% of all people. Although the typical single gene disorder is somewhat rare, their combined impact on human health is significant. In contrast, most common diseases are **multifactorial diseases**.

As the term "multifactorial" implies, there are multiple factors that can contribute to someone developing a multifactorial disease. We group these factors into two main categories: **genetic factors** and **nongenetic factors.** Some multifactorial diseases are caused primarily by genetic factors, while others are caused primarily by nongenetic factors. Most multifactorial diseases, however, result from a complex interaction between the specific variations the person has in his/her gene sequences (genetic factors) and his/her level of exposure to disease-causing agents that come to us through our diet, environment and lifestyle (nongenetic factors). This is a complicated, two-way interaction. Our genes and proteins interact with the things we come in contact with through our diet, environment and lifestyle, but the things we come in contact with through our diet, environment and lifestyle also influence the level of activity in our genes and proteins.

Once researchers turned their attention to multifactorial diseases, they began to explore the full range of variability in human DNA, and the full depth of human biology. As they went deeper into studying the variability in our genes and proteins, they also realised that, in order to include all the factors that cause disease in their studies, they would have to expand their focus beyond mere genetics.

RESEARCHERS HAVE HAD TO EXPAND THEIR FOCUS BEYOND GENETICS

The Human Genome Project Was A Race To The Starting Line, Not The Finish Line

The Human Genome Project (HGP) brought together researchers from the government, academia and private businesses, with the primary goal of discovering the sequence of human DNA. When the HGP published its first draft of the human DNA sequence in 2000, it was considered a landmark achievement.

Although this was a great accomplishment, it marked the beginning of an era of research, not the end of one. Having the sequence of a creature's DNA molecule is like discovering a library whose books are written in a language you have never seen before. You first need to learn the letters or characters that make up that language, then you need to learn how the different letters are put together to make words. After that, you need to learn how these words are combined to make meaningful sentences. Finally, you need to understand how sentences can be put together to construct complex ideas, integrate thoughts into propositions, teach new concepts, convey beliefs, make predictions, and do all the other things that we consider part of our uniquely human ability to use language.

In Chapter 2 we describe the structure of DNA, and describe the process whereby our genes make our proteins. For the purpose of this discussion, however, all you need to keep in mind is that DNA and RNA are made by chaining nucleotides together, and that each nucleotide contains a base, which is the important part of the nucleotide for our purposes. There are four bases in DNA: we call them A, C, G and T. RNA also uses A, C and G, but it uses a base we call U instead of T. When we discuss the sequence of our DNA or RNA, we are referring to the order of the A, C, G and T bases in the DNA, or the A, C, G and U bases in RNA.

Our genes and our proteins are written in two related languages. DNA and RNA use bases as the letters in their language. The main function of our genes (which are made of DNA) is to make our proteins. They do so by first making an RNA called messenger RNA (mRNA), which then provides your body instructions on how to make that specific gene's protein. Once the mRNA is made, your body's protein-making machinery "reads" the sequence of bases in the mRNA and "writes" a protein. It "reads" the bases in the mRNA three at a time. Each three-base group is called a **codon**, and each codon acts like a word in a sentence (*i.e.* in the language of mRNA, every word has three letters in it). Your body's protein-synthesising machinery "reads" the codons in the mRNA just as a translator would read the words in a sentence that was written in one language (bases). It then "writes" that gene's protein by chaining amino acids together, just as a translator would chain a set of words from the second language together to make a sentence in the new language.

Figures 1.1 and 1.2 illustrate the different levels at which we need to understand the languages of our DNA, mRNA and proteins in order to understand how our genes affect our health. For this example, we have chosen the sequence of the gene that makes oxytocin. Oxytocin is a hormone that has many functions, many of which are related to giving birth and the period shortly after. It promotes the contractions of the uterus that dispel the afterbirth, and promotes milk production and mother-infant bonding, among other functions. We chose oxytocin because it only contains nine amino acids, so we could show the entire coding sequence of the gene and amino acid sequence of the protein in a figure.

Discovering the sequence of a gene and its mRNA merely teaches us what the letters of the DNA language are, and allows us to see the order in which the letters are assembled to make that particular gene and its mRNA. Just as in language, however, it is the way in which the letters are arranged into specific words that gives the final product its specific function. Just as each word has its own meaning and is able to play a specific role in your effort to convey your thoughts, each amino acid has unique physical and chemical properties, and is capable of playing a specific, unique role in the structure and function of the protein (Figure 1.1). The specific sequence of words in a sentence gives that sentence its ability to convey a unique thought and have a specific significance in the context of the conversation. Similarly, the specific amino acids that get chained together to make that gene's protein are what gives that protein its unique function, and therefore its unique significance to your health.

The Bases In DNA And mRNA Act As Letters In Their Language

Oxytoxin mRNA Coding Sequence:
UGCUACAUCCAGAACUGCCCCCUGGGA

English Letters:
allpeopleshouldlivetogetherinpeace

↓

The mRNA Codons And Amino Acids In The Protein Act As Words In Their Language

UGC   UAC   AUC   CAG   AAC   UGC
cysteine-tyrosine-isoleucine-glutamine-asparagine-cysteine-

CCC   CUG   GGA
proline-leucine-glycine

allpeopleshouldlivetogetherinpeace → all people should live together in peace

Figure 1.1 The bases in DNA and mRNA are like the letters of the genetic language, while the mRNA codons and amino acids in the protein are like the words of the genetic/protein languages.

Figure 1.2 illustrates how the specific sequence of amino acids that are in a protein is critical for allowing that protein to perform its function, just as the specific sequence in which a set of words is arranged determines whether they make a sentence with a specific function. For any set of amino acids, you can join those amino acids in any one of many different specific sequences, but only one sequence will make that particular protein, with its characteristic function. Similarly, for any set of words, you can arrange the words in many different specific sequences, but only one sequence will convey the meaning that you want the sentence to convey.

If The mRNA Codons, Amino Acids Or Words Are Not Arranged In The Proper Sequence, They Do Not Make A Functional Protein/Sentence

Functional Oxytocin:
cysteine-tyrosine-isoleucine-glutamine-asparagine-cysteine-proline-leucine-glycine

Functional Sentence:
all people should live together in peace

Same Amino Acids, Difference Sequence, Not A Functional Protein:
tyrosine-glutamine-isoleucine-glycine-cysteine-proline-leucine-cysteine-asparagine

Same Words, Different Sequence, Not A Functional Sentence:
live peace should in together people all

Same Sequence Of mRNA Bases, But Organised Into Codons Differently, Does Not Make A Functional Protein:

U   GCU   ACA   UCC   AGA   ACU   GCC
    alanine-threonine-serine-arginine-threonine-alanine-

 CCC   UGG   GA
proline-tryptophan

Same Sequence Of Letters, But Organised Into Words Differently, Does Not Make A Functional Sentence:
allpe oplesho uld li vetoge th eri npea ce

Figure 1.2 The amino acids of a protein or the words of a sentence must be arranged in a specific sequence in order for that protein or sentence to perform its intended function.

The Field Of Genetics Has Expanded Into The Field Of Genomics

Researchers have come to understand a great deal about how the language of DNA is used to make our proteins. The focus of the early research was on genetics – the sequences of our genes, and how variations in a gene's sequence can affect your health. Once researchers began learning about the functions of our genes and proteins, however, it became clear that, in order to truly understand the significance that variations in gene sequences have for our health, it is necessary to understand how different genes and proteins interact with each other, and how our genes and proteins interact with nongenetic factors.

As researchers became more aware of how complex our genes' influence over our health is, the field of genetics expanded into the field of **genomics**. The term **genome** refers to a person's (or any life form's) entire DNA sequence, or the entire collection of genes that individual possesses. Genomic researchers don't just study the process whereby our genes make our proteins, they study the way our genes and proteins fit into the larger context of our metabolism. Genomic researchers study not only the way our genes and proteins process the things our bodies come into contact with through our diet, environment and lifestyle, but also how the things we come into contact with through our diet, environment and lifestyle affect the activity of our genes and proteins. As researchers have come to appreciate how many of these factors influence our health, and how complex their interactions are, another cornerstone principle of personalised medicine has emerged:

> Personalised medicine sees each person's body as an integrated ecosystem, with the different elements of the ecosystem (genetic, dietary, environmental, lifestyle, experience) influencing each other, and mechanisms in place to keep the different aspects of the ecosystem in balance with each other.

One of the most exciting areas in which new discoveries in personalised medicine are being made is that of nutrition and **epigenetics** (discussed in Chapter 7). Epigenetics refers to the fact that our DNA undergoes chemical reactions that do not change the sequence of bases in the gene, but change the rate at which the gene makes its protein. Genomic researchers have recently discovered that some of the things we consume (food, drink, prescription and recreational drugs) can influence this process, and thereby influence our health. They have even suggested that some of the things a pregnant woman consumes can change the level of activity in her baby's genes and proteins, thereby influencing the child's development and health.

Figure 1.3 illustrates the complex ways in which genetic, nongenetic and epigenetic factors influence each other. Note that these are two-way interactions. Your genes make your proteins, but some of your proteins also affect the activity level of your genes. Your proteins process many of the nongenetic factors you encounter through your diet, environment and lifestyle, but many of these nongenetic factors also influence the activity of your proteins. Nongenetic factors can influence the activity of genes in several ways, either directly or by influencing the epigenetic factors that influence the activity of your genes. One of the biggest challenges facing researchers in the field of personalised medicine today is determining exactly how the critical genetic, nongenetic and epigenetic factors interact to influence your risk for any given disease.

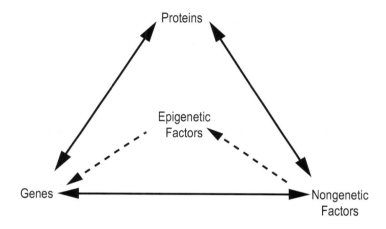

Figure 1.3 Genetic, nongenetic and epigenetic factors interact in complex ways to influence your risk for any given disease.

"GENETIC FACTORS" DETERMINE THE LEVELS OF ACTIVITY YOU HAVE IN YOUR PROTEINS

In order to understand how these "genetic factors" influence your health, you need to understand that your genes make your proteins, and your proteins do many of the jobs that must be done in order to keep you healthy. For example, they break down your food and deliver the nutrients to your body's cells, they battle the disease-causing bacteria and viruses you encounter in your environment, and they repair the damage that environmental factors such as smoking and the ultraviolet (UV) rays of the sun do to your body.

Chapter 2 describes the process by which a gene makes its protein, and provides specific examples of the way that variations in our genes' sequences can cause different people to have different levels of risk for specific diseases. For our present purposes, all you need to understand is that different people often have different versions of a given gene's sequence (each specific version of a gene's sequence is called an **allele** of that gene), and that some versions of the gene's sequence make versions of the protein that have different levels of activity than other versions of the protein have. This is another important cornerstone of personalised medicine:

> Because your proteins perform many of the functions that are required to keep you healthy, when different people have different levels of activity in specific proteins, they will also have different levels of risk for certain diseases.

You are probably familiar with the normal distribution, or "bell curve" depicted in Figure 1.4. If you measure almost any human trait in a large enough group of people, you will often get results that resemble the normal distribution. Most people have a value of that trait (such as height) that is close to the average. In addition, there are always people who differ from the average by a small margin, and a few people who fall well above or well below the average. If you measured the level of activity in most of our proteins in a large group of people, you would get a curve similar to the one in Figure 1.4.

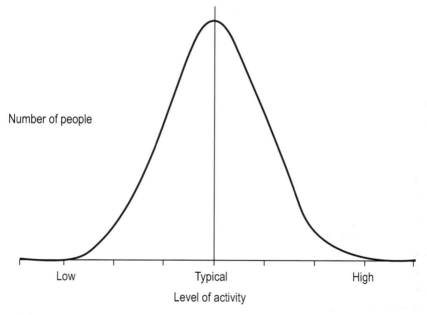

Figure 1.4 If you measure the level of activity in a protein in a large group of people, you get a range of values that approximates the normal distribution, or "bell curve."

To the extent that the function of that gene's protein influences your risk for a specific disease, if you drew a graph that depicted people's risks for that disease, the curve would also approximate the normal distribution. Because there are so many different factors that influence disease risk, many of which are still unrecognised, it is often impossible to give someone their exact probability of developing the disease of interest. More often, we group people according to whether they have a low, moderate or high risk of developing the disease compared to the typical person's risk. There are a few ways of quantifying the degree to which a risk-increasing or risk-decreasing allele influences your risk. These expressions all state your risk versus the typical person's risk, or they state the risk you have if you have one or two risk-increasing (or risk-decreasing) alleles compared to what your risk would be if you did not have any. For example, as we discuss in Chapter 6, the effect of a risk-increasing or risk-decreasing allele can be expressed as **relative risk** (RR). If a risk-increasing allele carries an RR of 2.0, for example, someone who has that risk-increasing allele has twice the risk of developing the disease in question than he/she would if he/she did not have that risk-increasing allele.

WE CANNOT AVOID MANY OF THE NONGENETIC FACTORS WE ENCOUNTER THROUGH OUR DIET, ENVIRONMENT AND LIFESTYLE

The average person gets exposed to a number of things that have the potential to make him/her sick every day. For example, you already know that picking up "germs" from other people can make you sick. You know that you pick up viruses and bacteria from other people every time you touch a door handle, or sit in a confined space with a group of people for any length of time (such as on an airplane). The only reason why you aren't constantly sick with a cold or the flu is the fact that your immune system proteins constantly fight these disease-causing agents, and prevent you from getting sick (or help you recover when you do). You can certainly choose living and working conditions that minimise your contact with other people. Because viruses and bacteria can spread through the air, and live on surfaces for hours or days, however, it is virtually impossible to avoid contacting other people's viruses and bacteria unless you live an extraordinarily secluded life.

There are many different environmental factors that can also impact our health. These include aspects of our internal environment as well as our external environment. For example, when your body breaks down (metabolises) the fat from the foods you eat, some of your body cells generate chemicals that are known as superoxide radicals, or reactive oxygen species. Superoxide radicals damage your arteries, and generating excessive amount of superoxide radicals increases your risk of developing heart disease. You can't avoid these superoxide radicals. Even if you eat a zero-fat diet, your body will metabolise your stored fat for energy, and make these superoxide radicals in the process. You can reduce your risk for heart disease by reducing the amount of fat in your diet, but you can never avoid this potential disease-causing agent altogether.

The UV rays of the sun are another nongenetic, disease-causing factor that you cannot avoid without taking extraordinary measures. As we mentioned above, the sun's UV rays can damage your DNA, and this can lead to skin cancer. You can certainly limit your exposure to the sun, but even walking in the sun with a bare head and arms for a short period of time causes damage to the DNA in your skin cells. Your DNA-repair proteins constantly work to repair this damage, but if you have low-activity versions of the DNA repair proteins, this process will not work as effectively in you as it does in other people. Like so many other nongenetic factors, you can reduce your level of exposure to the sun, or wear a high level SPF sunscreen, but you would have to take extraordinary measures to avoid it completely.

Some of the more preventable nongenetic causes of disease come from our lifestyles. Smoking, for example, contributes to a variety of respiratory (lung) diseases, several types of cancer and other diseases. Although it is easy to reduce your exposure to some of these lifestyle-related factors, it is still very difficult to avoid them altogether. It is usually easiest to see the effects of a nongenetic factor in someone who has exposed him/ herself to an extreme level of that factor (for example, lung cancer in someone who has smoked for many years). However, even a moderate amount of exposure to one of these nongenetic factors may carry some risk with it. Even occasional smoking or second hand smoke will expose you to disease-causing agents that your proteins must then protect you from.

The term "environmental factors" is often used to refer to the nongenetic factors that influence your risk of developing multifactorial diseases. "Nongenetic factors" is a better term, however, because these nongenetic factors include not only the things you encounter in your environment, but also the things that you expose yourself to through the choices you make about your diet and your lifestyle. The nongenetic factors that both increase and decrease your risk for a particular disease make up your **nongenetic load** for that disease.

YOUR GENETIC FACTORS INTERACT WITH NONGENETIC FACTORS TO INFLUENCE YOUR SUSCEPTIBILITY TO MULTIFACTORIAL DISEASES

Your proteins don't always protect you from diseases, however; some of your proteins actually create disease-causing agents. For example, the proteins that metabolise the fats you eat provide you with energy, but they also create chemicals called superoxide radicals. These superoxide radicals damage tissues, and can contribute to many different diseases.

Figures 1.5 and 1.6 illustrate the way in which genetic and nongenetic factors interact to influence your risk for atherosclerosis, or hardening of the arteries. As Figure 1.5

illustrates, some proteins protect you from disease-causing agents, while others create disease-causing agents. The proteins that digest the fats in your diet provide you with energy, but also create superoxide radicals, which can scar the linings of your arteries. Once that happens, the healing process causes fats to collect around the site of the scarring, and eventually block blood flow through that artery. You have other proteins that detoxify the superoxide radicals, however, and prevent them from scarring your arteries.

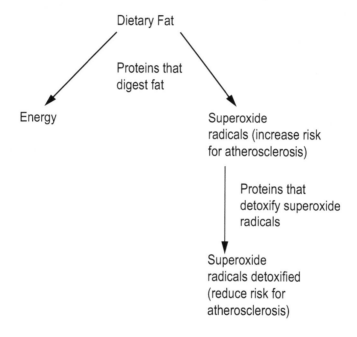

Figure 1.5 Some proteins create disease-causing agents, while others protect you from them.

Figure 1.6 illustrates the way in which some of your genetic and nongenetic factors interact to influence your risk for atherosclerosis. Beginning at the top of the figure, one nongenetic factor that will influence your risk is the level of fat in your diet. Going down from there, the level of activity in the enzymes that digest your fats will influence the amount of superoxide radicals your body makes. After that, the rate at which your body detoxifies these superoxide radicals is influenced by both the level of activity in the proteins that detoxify the superoxide radicals (genetic factors) and the level of antioxidants in your diet (a nongenetic factor). These factors influence the amount of scarring your arteries suffer, which in turn influences your risk for atherosclerosis.

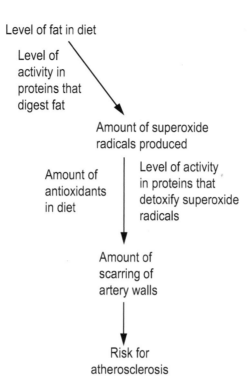

Figure 1.6 Several genetic and nongenetic factors interact to influence your risk for atherosclerosis.

Finally, we also need to understand how all the metabolic pathways in our bodies work together, to understand all the effects a particular genetic or nongenetic factor is going to have on our health. There is a great deal of feedback between your metabolic pathways; the products of one pathway often activate or inhibit activity in another pathway in order to keep all your systems in their proper balance. As our understanding of the complexity of the situation has grown, we have become aware that we need to expand the focus of research, to enable us to understand how our genes and their proteins interact with each other, with the other molecules in our bodies, and with nongenetic factors such as dietary factors or environmental toxins.

. . . .

A Quick Review Before We Move On

- Diseases can be classified as either single-gene diseases or multifactorial diseases. As the terms imply, single-gene diseases are caused by a mutation in a single gene, while the typical multifactorial disease has multiple potential causes. Many of the most common diseases people suffer from or are at risk for are multifactorial diseases.

- Some multifactorial diseases are caused primarily by genetic factors, while others are caused primarily by nongenetic factors. Most multifactorial diseases, however, are caused by a combination of genetic factors and nongenetic factors.

- The term "nongenetic factors" refers to the fact that we get exposed to a number of different things that can make us sick through our diet, environment and lifestyle. Some of these nongenetic factors are things we cannot avoid, even if we carefully monitor our diets, avoid dangerous environments and live a conservative lifestyle.

- The genetic factors that influence your risk for specific diseases come from the fact that different people often have slightly different versions of a given gene's sequence. This means that different people often have different levels of activity in the protein that gene makes. Your proteins perform many of the functions that are required to keep you healthy. If you have a level of activity in any given protein that is significantly greater than or less than that of the typical person, your risk for any diseases that protein's function influences will be greater or less than the typical person's risk.

- The genetic factors you are born with interact with the nongenetic factors you encounter throughout your life to determine your risk for the common multifactorial diseases. This is a complex, two-way interaction: your genes and proteins process the nongenetic factors you encounter, but the nongenetic factors you encounter also influence the activity of your genes and proteins.

· ·

The Field Of Personalised Medicine Holds Great Promise

Personalised Medicine Tests Will Increase Safety And Effectiveness While Reducing The Cost Of Healthcare

Personalising medicine has great potential to reduce the cost of healthcare while improving the safety and effectiveness of many people's treatments. Approximately 40-50% of people who are prescribed drugs do not improve. Worse yet, adverse drug reactions (ADRs) account for approximately 10-15% of emergency room admissions.

Until doctors have a better way of determining which drug and dose will be safest and most effective for each individual person, however, they will often be forced to begin with a standard first-line drug and dose, then engage in a potentially long trial-and-error process until they arrive at the right drug and dose for you. One goal of personalised medicine is to improve the safety and effectiveness of our prescription drugs, by allowing doctors to determine right away which drug and dose will be best for each patient, without going through the long trial-and-error process they often must go through now.

Personalised Medicine Will Enable You To Play A More Active Role In Maintaining Your Own Health

You've probably heard it said many times, in one way or another, that your health is your most precious possession. We all want to be healthy, and remain as healthy as possible as we go into our later years. One of the goals of personalised medicine is to provide you with information that enables you to take an active role in maintaining your own health.

The fact that nongenetic factors play an important role in your susceptibility to many common multifactorial diseases is good news, because it means that, in many cases, you may be able to reduce your risk for many of these common diseases by making health-conscious decisions regarding your diet, environment and lifestyle. Unfortunately, however, not all people will be able to significantly reduce their risk for every disease. If your **genetic load** (the sum of your risk-increasing and risk-decreasing gene alleles) for a particular disease is very heavy, there may be little you can do to reduce your overall risk of developing the disease by modifying your diet, environment or lifestyle.

Even having a heavy genetic load for a disease does not guarantee you will get the disease, however. If you do have such a heavy genetic load that there is little you can do to influence your risk of developing the disease by diet, environment and lifestyle adjustments, you may be still be able to benefit from more aggressive or earlier screening. Screening tests may help identify the disease at an earlier stage, where treatment can be more effective. A good example is having people with increased genetic risk for colon cancer undergo colonoscopies and other screening procedures at an earlier age than is recommended for the general population. Colon cancer develops from pre-cancerous polyps in the colon. By screening earlier or more often than is typically recommended, your doctors can detect and remove pre-cancerous polyps as they form. This can significantly decrease your risk of actually developing colon cancer.

Some Difficult Challenges Remain, But They Can All Be Overcome

The Human DNA Sequence Is Much More Variable Than We Thought It Was

Just as the Human Genome Project represented a starting point for genomic researchers, the human DNA sequence that was reported in 2000 by the Human Genome Project also turned out to be a starting point for understanding the "normal" sequence of human DNA, rather than a finish line. The original human DNA sequence was derived from a small handful of healthy volunteers' DNAs. The sequence that was originally published is called the **reference sequence**. Having a single sequence that everyone recognises as the standard reference sequence gives researchers from different laboratories a way to describe the variations they find in their subjects in a way that allows all other researchers to understand exactly what their subjects' sequences are. We cannot call the reference sequence the "normal" human DNA sequence, however. Once researchers sequenced a few healthy individuals, they discovered the fourth cornerstone principle of personalised medicine:

> There is no single "normal" human DNA sequence, nor is there even a single "normal" sequence for any gene. There are many different versions of the human DNA sequence, or of any given gene's sequence, that can be found in healthy people, and can therefore be called a "normal" sequence.

DNA sequencing allows analysts in laboratories to determine the sequence of a gene, or even your entire DNA sequence, base-by-base. The sequence of our DNA is so variable that sequencing is the only way to identify all the genetic factors an individual has that contribute to a disease. Fortunately, as we discuss below, the cost of DNA sequencing is dropping to levels that are allowing researchers to use sequencing more often to collect data on their subjects. Soon the cost of sequencing will be low enough that sequencing will be able to be used routinely to diagnose diseases and choose the safest and most effective treatments for people.

The 1,000 Genomes Project (TGP www.1000genomes.org) is one of several large studies that are attempting to obtain the entire DNA sequence, and complete lifelong health information, from a large number of volunteers (in this case, 1,000). This group has recently reported preliminary results after obtaining the complete sequence of 179 different individuals from four different ethnic groups, including two mother-father-child "trios" (family units). They also sequenced critical portions of all the known (22,000-23,000) genes in almost 700 additional volunteers from seven different ethnic groups. According to the TGP report:

- If you compare the typical person's DNA sequence against the reference human DNA sequence, there are approximately 10,000-11,000 places at which you can find alterations in the DNA sequence that are expected to change the level of activity in one of our proteins.
- There are also 10,000–12,000 places at which you can find alterations in the DNA sequence that are not expected to change the level of activity in one of our proteins. In all likelihood, however, as we learn more about the factors that influence the activity of our proteins, some of those DNA sequence changes will be shown to influence a protein's activity.

- There are approximately 15 million places in the DNA sequence where some people have one base (*e.g.* an A), and other people have a different base (*e.g.* a C, G or T).
- There are approximately 1 million places in the typical person's DNA sequence where there is a short stretch of DNA that has been either added in or taken out, compared to the reference human DNA sequence.
- They found 20,000 larger structural variants in the DNA of these subjects. These structural variants involve situations in which a chromosome (we will discuss the makeup of a chromosome in Chapter 2) has lost material, gained material, had some material rearranged, or exchanged material with another chromosome. There are already many of these types of chromosome rearrangements that have been reported to occur, but most of the chromosome rearrangements the TGP reported had not been reported before.
- The typical person has approximately 50 to 100 sequence changes that are thought to be capable of causing a genetic disease if both copies of the gene had that sequence (*i.e.* recessive disease-causing mutations, discussed in Chapter 3).
- The typical person has a surprising number of DNA sequence variants that are expected to significantly reduce the level of activity in a protein. The list includes:
  190–210 insertions or deletions in a gene's coding sequence
  80–100 changes in a gene's coding sequence that will cause the cell to stop making the protein before it has been completed
  220–250 deletions that cause the cell to put the wrong amino acid building blocks into the protein
- When parents pass their DNA down to their children, it is typical for approximately 30-35 single base changes (new mutations) to occur in the DNA sequence as it is passed from the parent to the child.

Although it is obvious that our DNA sequence is highly variable, researchers are now able to sequence genes to determine the full range of variability in our genes' sequences. It is merely a matter of time (and some hard work) before this information gets turned into tests that can help improve your healthcare.

Most Personalised Medicine Tests Will Have To Include Information About Many Genes

No protein works by itself. Your body's metabolism is organised into pathways. Each metabolic pathway is a series of biochemical reactions, each of which is run by a different enzyme (enzymes are proteins that run biochemical reactions). Each metabolic pathway accomplishes a goal, such as harvesting energy from your blood sugar, or assembling the protein hemoglobin so it can carry oxygen to your tissues. In order to assess all the factors that influence the function of any one metabolic pathway, and thereby influence your risk for whatever diseases involve that pathway, the analyst must gather information on dozens, or even hundreds, of genes.

The genetic factors we have discovered so far account for only a small percentage of the genetic factors that influence disease, or for that matter, our other multifactorial traits. For example, in 2007 a study that looked for genes that influenced height identified a dozen such genes. Together, these genes only accounted for approximately 2% of the variability in people's heights. Someone who had "tall" versions of all these genes was only, on average, one inch taller than someone who had "short" versions of all these genes. Similarly, in a recent study of 6,000 children, the gene with the biggest effect on the child's intelligence quotient (IQ) accounted for less than one-quarter of a point.

It is clear that, for many multifactorial traits and diseases, a test will have to assess the person's status for hundreds, perhaps even thousands, of genes to produce an accurate estimate of his/her risk for the trait or disease in question. Fortunately, DNA analysis technology has developed to a point where analysts can use microarrays (discussed in Chapter 5) to determine your status at hundreds of thousands of places in your DNA in one test, or whole-DNA sequencing to determine the sequence of every one of your genes at once.

One of the other big challenges to the development of personalised medicine is the challenge of properly interpreting the huge amount of information that modern-day DNA analyses can produce. Computer programs that enable analysts to interpret massive amounts of data are being developed, and will improve over time. As the amount of information an analyst can collect at one time grows, the ability to analyse and interpret this information effectively is growing as well.

Genetic And Nongenetic Factors Interact In Complex Ways

As we discussed above, one of the biggest challenges that researchers who are trying to develop personalised medicine tests face is the fact that there are many different ways in which genetic and nongenetic factors interact among themselves and with each other. In some cases, the risk-increasing and risk-reducing factors add up to determine your overall risk for a disease. In other cases, however, the effects of two factors can multiply when both factors are present, or even interact in a more dramatic manner than that.

For example, consider the toxicology (toxicology = the study of poisons) studies that have shown the interaction between lead and mercury. If you inject mice with a dose of lead that, by itself, would kill only 1% of the mice, and you then add a dose of mercury that, by itself, would also kill only 1% of the mice, all your mice will die. Lead and mercury interact **synergistically**, meaning that their combined effect is far greater than just adding together or even multiplying each other. Similarly, if you have low-activity or high-activity versions of two proteins that work together to protect you from a particular disease, their effects may add together, multiply each other, or combine synergistically.

Another complication that researchers have recently begun to appreciate is the fact that epigenetic factors have a strong influence on the activity of many of our genes. As we mentioned above, epigenetic factors influence the rate at which a gene produces its protein, which in turn influences the level of activity you have in that protein. As we discuss in Chapter 7, not only do our genes and proteins process the things we eat and drink, but the things we eat and drink can also influence the level of activity we have in our genes and proteins.

Both Your Nongenetic Load And Your Genetic Load May Increase As You Get Older

One of the biggest challenges that face researchers who are trying to develop personalised medicine tests is the fact that the status of specific genetic, epigenetic and nongenetic factors may change as you get older. For example, consider the disease hemochromatosis. Hemochromatosis results from having an excess of iron accumulate in your vital organs over a long period of time. As you age, the iron level in your body increases, and as it does, your risk for hemochromatosis increases as well.

It is easy to imagine that a nongenetic factor such as the level of iron in your body could increase over time. It is harder to understand how your genetic load can increase over time, but the fact is, it can as well. In Chapter 3, where we discuss the inheritance of genetic factors through the generations, we also discuss the concepts of **somatic mutations** and **mitochondrial DNA mutations**. Somatic mutations and mitochondrial DNA mutations can contribute to a great many diseases. One of the challenges personalised medicine researchers face when they try to assemble all the critical factors into a formula that predicts your risk for a certain disease is the fact that your status regarding somatic mutations and mitochondrial DNA mutations changes as you get older.

The Pace Of Discovery Has Increased Impressively For The Past Few Decades

Over the past few decades, several genetic testing technologies have been developed that enable researchers to collect and interpret enormous amounts of data. Microarrays, or "gene chips" (discussed in Chapter 5), have been developed that enable researchers to assess the individual's sequence at hundreds of thousands, even millions, of places in the DNA in one assay. In addition, the cost of microarray analyses and DNA sequencing DNA is rapidly decreasing, and will soon drop to a level at which it will become feasible to routinely obtain a person's entire DNA sequence.

As Figure 1.7 illustrates, the cost of sequencing DNA has declined steadily in the last 15 years. As the cost of sequencing has declined, the amount of sequence information that is being generated each year has risen just as dramatically. With 3.3 billion base pairs in the human DNA sequence, at 1990's cost of $10 per basepair, sequencing a person's entire DNA molecule cost 33 billion dollars ($33,000,000,000). As you can see from the figure, however, the cost of sequencing has decreased steadily since then, and this has greatly increased the pace at which genomic researchers have been generating sequence data.

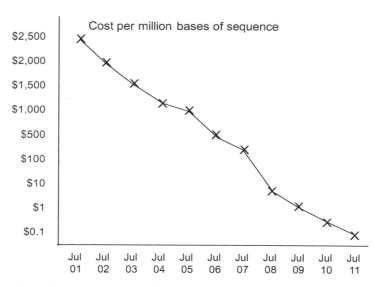

Figure 1.7 As the cost of sequencing has decreased in recent years, the pace at which researchers are generating sequence data has increased. From the U.S. Department of Energy Genome Programs, http://genomics.energy.gov.

THIS BOOK WILL HELP YOU GET THE MAXIMUM BENEFIT FROM THESE NEW ADVANCES

Your genes and proteins impact every aspect of your health, and the principles discussed in this book will someday touch every aspect of medicine. In the not too distant future, personalised medicine tests will become a routine part of everyone's healthcare. In the meantime, this book will help you understand the potential benefits, as well as the limitations, of these newly developed genetic tests. This book will help you better understand what genetic tests are available right now, and what information can and cannot be obtained from them.

In addition, this book will also help you better understand how to use your family's medical history and programs you can access on the internet to estimate your risk for the diseases that run in your family. Most primary-care doctors' office visits are so short that the doctor doesn't have time to collect extensive family history data. In Chapter 4, we show you some Internet sites that can help you draw up your family's pedigree (family tree), so you can collect your family's health information and present it to your doctor in a manner that enables him/her to determine the implications your family history has for your care.

CHAPTER SUMMARY

- Many of the most common diseases people suffer from or are at risk for are multifactorial diseases. Some multifactorial diseases are caused primarily by genetic factors, while others are caused primarily by nongenetic factors. Most multifactorial diseases, however, are caused by a combination of genetic factors and nongenetic factors.

- The term "nongenetic factors" refers to the fact that we get exposed to a number of different things that can make us sick through our diet, environment and lifestyle. Some of these nongenetic factors are things we cannot avoid, even if we carefully monitor our diets, avoid dangerous environments and live a conservative lifestyle.

- The genetic factors that influence your risk for specific diseases come from the fact that different people often have slightly different versions of a given gene's sequence. This means that different people often have different levels of activity in the protein that gene makes. Because your proteins perform many of the functions that are required to keep you healthy, if you have a level of activity in any given protein that is significantly greater than or less than that of the typical person, your risk for any diseases that protein's function influences will be greater or less than the typical person's risk.

- The genetic factors you are born with interact with the nongenetic factors you encounter throughout your life to determine your risk for the common multifactorial diseases. This is a complex, two-way interaction: your genes and proteins process the nongenetic factors you encounter, but the nongenetic factors you encounter also influence the activity of your genes and proteins.

- Personalised medicine tests will enable your doctor to prescribe the safest and most effective treatments for you. They will greatly reduce the amount of time and money that is wasted when people get prescribed drugs that do not work, and will reduce the frequency with which people suffer dangerous side effects from drugs.

- Personalised medicine tests are being developed that will reveal whether you have any variations in your gene sequences that increase or decrease your risk for specific diseases, and help your doctor more accurately estimate your risk for developing certain diseases. People who have light to moderate genetic loads may be able to reduce their risk of developing a particular multifactorial disease by adjusting their diet, environment and lifestyle to minimise their exposure to the critical nongenetic factors. Even those who have heavy genetic loads, however, may be able to reduce their risk of developing the disease, or reduce its impact on their lives, by undergoing more frequent or more intensive screening procedures to detect the disease at a time when there is a better chance of treating or curing it.

- One of the important challenges facing personalised medicine researchers is the fact that it will often be necessary to combine an assessment of hundreds of different genetic and nongenetic factors in order to produce the best possible estimate of someone's risk for a specific disease. Fortunately, DNA analysis technology has developed to the point where it is possible to collect such huge amounts of information. In addition, computer programs that enable analysts to interpret this mass of information effectively have been developed and are being improved.

- One of the other big challenges to the researchers who are trying to develop personalised medicine tests that can help predict your risk for specific diseases is to determine exactly how the different factors that influence your risk for a given disease interact. Some may add up when combined, but others may multiply each other, or even interact more dramatically than that.

- In addition, the best personalised medicine tests will take into account the fact that the degree to which genetic factors and nongenetic factors influence your risk for a specific disease may change over the course of your life.

- The speed at which new discoveries are being made is increasing all the time. Personalised medicine will soon impact a great many fields of medicine. This book can help you get the maximum benefit from these new advances in healthcare.

CHAPTER 2

THE MECHANISM WHEREBY A GENE MAKES ITS PROTEIN

Your genes make your proteins, and your proteins perform many of the functions that are required for you to remain healthy. This means that, in order to understand the means by which your genes influence your health, you need to know a little bit about the process by which your genes make your proteins. In this chapter, we present the essential details of this process[1]. Understanding this material will enable you to understand how testing one of your gene's sequences can give you information about your risk for a specific disease, or about your risk for a dangerous side effect from a given prescription drug. It will enable you to understand not only what information the new genetic tests will provide, but also the limitations of that information.

As you read through this chapter, keep the following overview in mind:

- Your genes make your proteins, and your proteins perform many of the functions that are required to keep you healthy. Your proteins all need to work at certain levels of activity in order to maintain your health.
- A protein is made by chaining amino acids together. There are 20 amino acids that are used to make your proteins. Each amino acid has a unique chemical structure. Some are positively charged, others are negatively charged and some are electrically neutral. The sequence of a gene determines which amino acids will be chained together to make that gene's protein.
- In order for a protein to perform its function, and to work at the proper level of activity, it must be able to adopt its characteristic three-dimensional (3D) shape, and to move to some degree as it works. If the sequence of the gene changes, this sometimes (but not always) changes the sequence of amino acids in the gene's protein. If the sequence of amino acids in the protein changes, this may change the protein's 3D shape or its ability to move. This may reduce, completely do away with, or even increase the protein's level of activity.
- The genetic factors that influence your risk for specific diseases come from the fact that the sequence of a typical gene is highly variable. Different people often

---

[1]   We have deliberately omitted some details, and condensed some multi-step processes into one step, to focus on the important aspects of the process, and avoid introducing too many technical terms.

have slightly different versions of a given gene's sequence. This means that different people often have different levels of activity in the protein that gene makes. Because your proteins perform many of the functions that are required to keep you healthy, if you have a level of activity in any given protein that is significantly greater than or less than that of the typical person, your risk for any diseases that protein's function influences will be greater or less than the typical person's risk.

Although we provide several figures to help you understand this material, still figures often cannot demonstrate a dynamic process like this as well as videos. To view the current Internet videos that illustrate this process, search for videos depicting **transcription** (the process whereby the DNA is used to make the mRNA) and **translation** (the process whereby the mRNA is used to make the protein).

THE PROCESS HAS TWO MAJOR STEPS

You don't need to understand all of the details of the process whereby a gene makes a protein to understand how your genes affect your health. In this section we present just the material you need to understand in order to understand why different versions of a gene's sequence may provide different levels of risk for a specific disease. In addition, understanding the way in which your genes make your proteins will help you understand what genetic tests actually look at, and why these tests can provide useful information regarding the level of activity in some of your proteins. Don't get bogged down in the details. Keep this overview in mind:

- DNA is made by chaining **nucleotides** together; each nucleotide has a component in it called a base. There are four different bases in the DNA nucleotides: you can call them A, C, G and T. For each gene, the sequence of bases in the gene determines the specific amino acids that get chained together to make that gene's protein.
- In the first step of the process, the sequence of bases in the gene provides the instructions to make the gene's messenger RNA (mRNA). Like the DNA, the mRNA is also made of nucleotides, but the T base you find in DNA is replaced by another base, called U, in the mRNA.
- In the second step of the process, the sequence of bases in the mRNA determines the sequence of amino acids that get chained together to make the protein. There are 20 amino acids that are used to make your proteins, and each amino acid has a unique chemical structure.

THE STRUCTURE OF DNA

Figure 2.1 is intended to help you picture the structure of the DNA molecule. You've no doubt heard the term "double helix" used to describe the structure of your DNA molecule. You may not have heard the term "nucleotide," however, but nucleotides are the building blocks of your DNA (Figure 2.1 A).

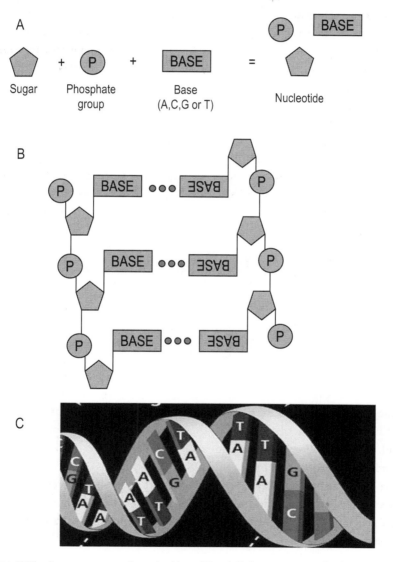

Figure 2.1 A) The three components of a nucleotide, and B and C) the arrangement whereby nucleotides are joined together to make the DNA double helix. Panel C is from the US Department of Energy Genomes Program, http://genomics.energy.gov

As panel A in Figure 2.1 illustrates, each nucleotide is made up of three components: the sugar deoxyribose[2] (shown as a pentagon), a phosphate group (shown as a circle with the letter "P" inside) and a base. There are four different types of nucleotides in DNA; each one contains a different base. Some nucleotides contain the base adenine (A), some contain the base cytosine (C), some contain the base guanine (G) and others contain the base thymine (T).

Panels B and C in Figure 2.1 shows how the nucleotides are chained together to make a strand of DNA, and how two DNA strands are bonded together to make the DNA double helix. One way to visualise the structure of DNA is to imagine taking an extension ladder and twisting it into a spiral. The handrails of the ladder represent the alternating sugar-phosphate group-sugar-phosphate group that make up the backbone of the double helix, while the footrungs of the ladder represent the bases, which project inward from the backbones. Bonds between the bases hold the two DNA strands together (shown as dotted lines between the bases). Because of the nucleotides' chemical structures, when you line up two strands of nucleotides, the complex adopts a helical structure (Figure 2.1 C).

For our purposes, the base is the most important part of the nucleotide. The sequence of bases in the gene determines which amino acids will be chained together to make the gene's protein. In turn, the sequence of amino acids in the protein determines the function the protein can perform, as well as the level of activity at which the protein works.

THE SEQUENCE OF BASES IN THE GENE'S CODING SEQUENCE DETERMINES THE SEQUENCE OF BASES IN THE GENE'S mRNA

When a gene makes its protein, the first thing that happens is the bonds between the bases are broken, separating the two strands of DNA, and the DNA double helix opens like a zipper. This produces two single strands of nucleotides, with the bases of the nucleotides exposed, like the teeth of the open zipper. Specialised proteins read the sequence of bases in one of the two DNA strands (*i.e.* they read the gene's **coding sequence**), and make a new molecule known as messenger RNA (mRNA).

The mRNA is also made up of nucleotides. As is true for DNA, the bases are the most important parts of the mRNA nucleotides as well; the sequence of bases in the gene's mRNA will determine the sequence of amino acids that get chained together to make that gene's protein. The sequence of bases in the gene's mRNA is identical to the

---

2   The fact that deoxyribose is the sugar in DNA nucleotides gives DNA its formal name deoxyribonucleic acid.

sequence of bases in the gene's coding sequence, except the mRNA nucleotides contain the base uracil (U) where the DNA nucleotides contains thymine (T). For example:

If the gene's coding sequence is: ATCCATGCTA
The corresponding mRNA sequence is: AUCCAUGCUA

The process whereby the DNA is used to make the mRNA is called **transcription**. The process of transcription is similar to the process you would go through if you were asked to decorate a room for a party, given a string of lights with empty light sockets, a bucket with four different colored light bulbs in it, and a set of written instructions telling you to put the different colored light bulbs in their sockets in a specific sequence. Each time you added a light bulb to the string, you would read the instructions, choose from among the four different colored bulbs, and put the appropriately colored light bulb into the next open socket in the string. In the case of the gene making its mRNA, the cell has specialised proteins that read the bases in the DNA and use that information as instructions to chain the appropriate mRNA nucleotides together in the proper order. Each time they add a new nucleotide to the mRNA, these proteins choose the appropriate nucleotide from the four different mRNA nucleotides that are present in the cell, just as you would choose your next light bulb from among the four different colored light bulbs in your bucket.

THE SEQUENCE OF BASES IN THE GENE'S mRNA DETERMINES THE SEQUENCE OF AMINO ACIDS IN THE PROTEIN

To make a protein, one of the cell's many specialised machines, called a **ribosome**, reads the sequence of bases in the gene's mRNA and uses that as its instructions to chain together the appropriate amino acids. The process is known as **translation**, because the ribosome "reads" a mRNA that is "written" in bases, and "writes" a protein that is "written" in amino acids. The process of translation is similar to the process we described above, in which you were asked to decorate a room with a string of colored lights, and given instructions regarding the sequence in which the different colored lights should be strung. This time, however, there are 20 different amino acids that are used to make your proteins, so instead of four different colored light bulbs in the bucket, you have 20. Apart from that, the process is the same. The sequence of bases in the gene's mRNA acts like your written instructions, specifying the sequence of amino acids to be chained together. The ribosome chains together the amino acids, just as you would insert the light bulbs into the sockets in the specified order. Some proteins are short (10 amino acids in length), while other proteins are long (thousands of amino acids in length).

The ribosome reads the gene's mRNA three bases at a time. Each set of three bases is called a **codon**. Each codon instructs the ribosome to insert one amino acid into the growing chain. Because there are three nucleotides in a codon, and four possible nucleotides in each of those three positions, there are 64 possible mRNA codons (4 X 4 X 4 = 64).

Figure 2.2 illustrates the **genetic code**, i.e. the relationship between the base sequence in the mRNA codon and the amino acid that gets incorporated into the protein. As the table shows, when the ribosome reads a CAG codon, it incorporates the amino acid glutamine into the protein. When the ribosome reads an AUU codon, however, it incorporates the amino acid isoleucine into the protein. Notice also that three of the codons are STOP codons. When the ribosome reads a codon with the sequence UGA, UAG or UAA, it stops chaining amino acids together, and releases the chain of amino acids so it can be processed into the protein's final form, to be used by the cell.

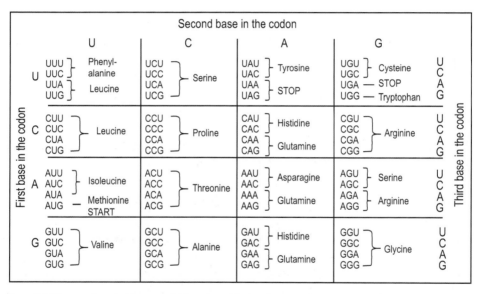

Figure 2.2 The genetic code illustrates which amino acids the ribosome incorporates into the protein when it reads each of the 64 different possible mRNA codons.

Let's look at an example, in which a portion of the gene's coding sequence is GTGCTAGCTTGA:

Gene's coding sequence	GTGCTAGCTTGA
Corresponding mRNA sequence	GUGCUAGCUUGA
mRNA codons	GUG CUA GCU UGA
Amino acids chained together	valine leucine alanine STOP

As you can see, the mRNA's base sequence is identical to the gene's coding sequence, except the mRNA has Us where the gene (DNA) has Ts. The mRNA is read in three-nucleotide codons, each of which directs the ribosome to add an amino acid into the protein. The UGA codon is one of the STOP codons; it directs the ribosome to stop chaining amino acids together. If this was the gene's entire coding sequence, the protein would consist of three amino acids: valine—leucine—alanine.

. . . .

A QUICK REVIEW BEFORE WE MOVE ON

- The sequence of bases in a gene determines the sequence of bases that gene's mRNA. The sequence of bases in the mRNA is identical to the sequence of bases in the gene's coding sequence, except mRNA uses the base uracil (U) where DNA uses the base thymine (T).
- The sequence of bases in the gene's mRNA determines the sequence of amino acids that get chained together to make that gene's protein. The genetic code allows you to read a mRNA's sequence and predict which amino acids will be chained together to make that gene's protein.

. . . .

DIFFERENT PEOPLE OFTEN HAVE SLIGHTLY DIFFERENT GENE SEQUENCES, WHICH MAY RESULT IN THEM HAVING DIFFERENT LEVELS OF ACTIVITY IN THEIR PROTEINS

The Sequence Of Bases In A Typical Gene Is Highly Variable

We all know that human biological traits are highly variable. If you look at any group of people, you can see that everyone has a unique combination of height, hair color, skin tone and eye color. Once scientists began sequencing people's DNA, they quickly learned that the sequence of our DNA is just as variable as our other traits. There is no single "normal" human DNA sequence. In fact, there isn't even a single "normal" sequence for any of our genes. For the typical gene, there are many different specific versions of the gene's sequence in the human population. Most of them can be considered "normal" sequences, because they enable the gene to make a version of the protein that has a level of activity that supports normal development and function.

Each of the different versions of a gene's sequence that exists in the population is called an **allele** of that gene. In most cases, the specific difference between one allele's sequence and another allele's sequence is minor—perhaps even as small as one single base change. As the example we provide at the end of this section illustrates, however, even a single base change in a gene's sequence can significantly alter the level of activity in that gene's protein.

Changing The Base Sequence In A Gene Sometimes Changes The Level Of Activity In That Gene's Protein

When two different people have slightly different versions of a gene's sequence, this may or may not result in them having a slightly different sequence of amino acids in that gene's protein. For example, imagine that the four sequences in Figure 2.3 represent four different alleles of a gene. As you can see from the figure, there is only one base difference between Alexandra's sequence and any of the other three sequences. Ben has a T where Alexandra has an A, Shannon has a C where Alexandra has a G, and Dustin has an A where Alexandra has a G. Let's imagine that Alexandra's allele is the most common allele that exists in the population, and it makes a version of the protein that has a typical level of activity.

Figure 2.3 illustrates the differences between the four people in terms of what their mRNA sequences will be, and what three-base codons the ribosome will read when it reads the mRNA. It also illustrates that not all changes in the coding sequence of the gene cause a change in the amino acid sequence of the protein. You can see that, while Ben's mRNA sequence is different from Alexandra's, the sequence of amino acids in his protein is not. If you go back to the genetic code table in Figure 2.2, you can see that the genetic code is partially redundant; there are many cases in which more than one codon will instruct the ribosome to incorporate the same amino acid into the protein. In Ben's case, his GGU codon instructed his ribosomes to incorporate glycine into the protein, just as Alexandra's GGA codon instructed her ribosomes to do. Because there is no difference in the sequence of the amino acids in Alexandra's and Ben's proteins, their proteins will have the same level of activity. To the extent that this protein influences your risk for specific diseases, their risks will be the same.

In contrast, you can see from Figure 2.3 that the amino acid sequence of Shannon's and Dustin's proteins are slightly different from Alexandra's and Ben's. Shannon has the amino acid alanine where Alexandra and Ben have glycine, while Dustin has the amino acid arginine in that position. You can also see from the figure that glycine, alanine and arginine have different chemical structures. The boxes illustrate the differences between them; alanine is just a little larger than glycine, while arginine is considerably larger than glycine. In addition, arginine has a positive electrical charge, while glycine and alanine are uncharged.

Coding sequence	mRNA sequence
Alexandra CTA**GGA**TGC	CUA**GGA**UGC
Ben CTA**GGT**TGC	CUA**GGU**UGC
Shannon CTA**GCA**TGC	CUA**GCA**UGC
Dustin CTA**AGA**TGC	CUA**AGA**UGC

mRNA codons	Amino acid sequence
Alexandra CUA, **GGA**, UGC	leucine, **glycine**, cysteine
Ben CUA, **GGU**, UGC	leucine, **glycine**, cysteine
Shannon CUA, **GCA**, UGC	leucine, **alanine**, cysteine
Dustin CUA, **AGA**, UGC	leucine, **arginine**, cysteine

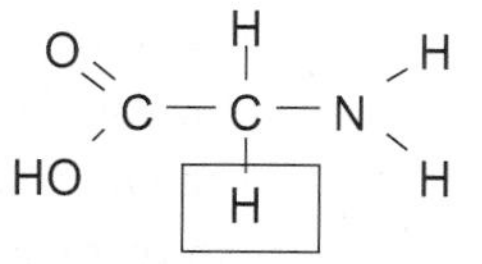

Glycine—small, uncharged

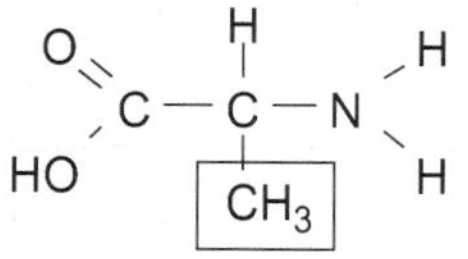

Alanine—small, uncharged

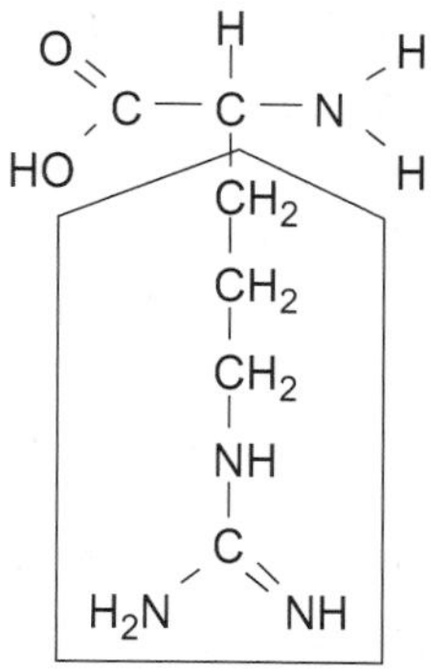

Arginine—large, positively charged

Figure 2.3 Four different alleles of a hypothetical gene's sequence, and the resultant differences in the amino acid content of the corresponding protein.

In order to function properly, and to have the necessary level of activity, a protein must be able to fold into its proper 3D shape, and to move and change shape to some degree as it performs its function. Anything that changes the protein's ability to adopt its characteristic 3D shape, or to move as it needs to while it performs its function, will change the level of activity at which the protein works.

The protein's 3D shape is maintained by a number of forces, including the fact that amino acids with opposite charges will attract each other, and amino acids with similar charges will repel each other. If a change in the gene's sequence causes one amino acid to be substituted by an amino acid with a different electrical charge, this may prevent the protein from folding into its 3D shape. Similarly, the protein's ability to bend depends on having certain amino acids at the flex points. If a change in the gene's sequence causes a small amino acid that sits at a flex point in the protein to be substituted for by a larger amino acid, or one that does not bend as easily, the protein may not be able to move as it needs to.

In Shannon's case, alanine is just a little larger than glycine, and like glycine, has no electrical charge. Substituting alanine in for glycine will probably not change the protein's ability to fold into its 3D shape and move as it needs to, and therefore will probably not affect the activity of the protein very much. To the extent that this protein influences your risk for specific diseases, Shannon's risk will be very similar to Alexandra's and Ben's.

As Figure 2.3 illustrates, Dustin has the amino acid arginine in this position in his protein. Unlike glycine and alanine, arginine is large and positively charged. This may seriously interfere with the protein's ability to fold into its 3D shape and move as it needs to in order to perform its function.

Risk-Increasing Versus Risk-Decreasing Alleles

The most important way to categorise the different alleles of a gene is by whether they increase or decrease your risk for the corresponding disease. Some authors call the alleles that increase your susceptibility to a disease "high-risk" alleles for that disease, and the alleles that decrease your susceptibility to a disease "low-risk" alleles. We, however, prefer to refer to gene alleles as **typical-risk alleles**, **risk-increasing alleles** or **risk-decreasing alleles**.

We feel that the use of the terms "high-risk" and "low-risk" make people think that if they have a "high-risk" allele for a disease, they have a high overall risk for that disease. This is misleading. Because the typical multifactorial disease requires several genetic and nongenetic factors to combine before the person develops the disease, many risk-increasing alleles only increase your overall risk for the disease by a small amount. Someone who has a "high-risk" allele, but no other significant genetic or nongenetic factors, may have a low overall risk for developing the disease. Similarly, someone who has a protective, "low-risk" allele of one critical gene, but has significant other genetic and nongenetic factors, may have a high overall risk for the disease.

Whether a given gene allele will be a typical-risk allele, a risk-increasing allele or a risk-decreasing allele depends on what the function of that gene's protein is, and whether that gene allele increases or decreases the protein's level of activity compared to the typical person's level of activity. As we discussed in Chapter 1, some of your proteins actually create disease-causing agents (*e.g.* the proteins that carry out the normal process of breaking down fat in your body produce superoxide radicals that promote atherosclerosis, or hardening of the arteries). If the protein generates the disease-causing agent, having a high-activity version of that protein increases your risk for the disease, while having a low-activity version of the protein provides you a little extra protection from the disease. The alleles of the gene that make the high-activity versions of the protein are considered risk-increasing alleles, while the alleles of the gene that make the low-activity versions of the protein are therefore considered the risk-decreasing alleles.

In other cases, your proteins protect you against one or more nongenetic factors that can make you sick (*e.g.* proteins that prevent cancer by repairing the damage the sun's UV rays do to your skin cells' DNA). For these proteins, having a high-activity version of the protein provides you a little extra protection from that disease, while having a low-activity version of the protein increases your risk. In this case, the alleles of the gene that make the low-activity versions of the protein are considered risk-increasing alleles, while the alleles of the gene that make the high-activity versions of the protein are considered risk-decreasing alleles.

For the proteins that influence your susceptibility to a particular multifactorial disease, the combination of high-risk and low-risk alleles you possess for the associated genes make up your genetic factors, or **genetic load**, for that particular disease. These genetic factors interact, sometimes in complex ways, with certain nongenetic factors that you encounter through your diet, environment and lifestyle to determine your overall risk of developing the disease.

Even Small Differences In A Gene's Sequence Can Significantly Change The Level Of Activity In The Gene's Protein

In many cases, the difference between two people's gene sequences is very small, but the difference in the level of activity of that protein can be significant. In fact, the most common variant we know of is the **single nucleotide polymorphism** (abbreviated **SNP**, pronounced "snip"). The word **polymorphism** comes from the Latin roots poly (many) and morph (form). Any characteristic that differs between different people is a polymorphic trait. This includes physical characteristics such as the shape of your earlobe, personality traits such as your level of optimism, medical characteristics such as your level of susceptibility to a specific disease, or a genetic trait such as the possession of a C versus an A nucleotide at one spot in a gene's coding sequence. A SNP, as the name implies, involves one single nucleotide in a gene's coding sequence. Some people will have one base (*e.g.* an A) at that position in the DNA, while other people will have a different base (*e.g.* a C, G or T) in that spot. In spite of the fact that this represents a tiny change in a gene's sequence, SNPs can have significant effects on the activity level of the protein. There are at least 15 million SNPs in the human DNA sequence. Many of them influence the level of activity of a gene or its protein.

Figure 2.4 illustrates how a SNP in the *HFE* gene[3] influences your susceptibility to hemochromatosis. Hemochromatosis results from the accumulation of excessive levels of iron in the body over time. The symptoms of hemochromatosis include abdominal pain, weakness, fatigue, darkening of the skin, joint pain, lack of energy, loss of body hair and loss of sexual desire. Because it usually takes several decades before enough iron accumulates to cause the person to feel its effects, hemochromatosis usually develops around middle age. There are several nongenetic factors that influence your risk for hemochromatosis, including the level of iron in your diet, and whether you are male or female[4]. These nongenetic factors interact with several genetic factors to determine your overall risk for hemochromatosis. The HFE protein helps regulate the level of iron in your body, so any sequence variation that changes the level of activity in the HFE protein can alter your risk for hemochromatosis.

For this SNP, most people have the G base at base number 845 in the gene's coding sequence[5], while others have the A base. Recall from earlier in this chapter that the ribosome reads the gene's mRNA three nucleotides at a time, and each three-nucleotide codon instructs the ribosome to add one amino acid to the protein. Because of this 3:1 arrangement, base 845 is the second base in codon 282 (282 X 3 = 846).

As Figure 2.4 illustrates, the sequence of the 282nd codon in the G allele of the *HFE* gene is TGC (UGC in the mRNA), which instructs the ribosome to add the amino acid cysteine in as the 282nd amino acid in the *HFE* protein. The 282nd codon's sequence in the A allele of the *HFE* gene is TAC (UAC in the mRNA), which causes the ribosome to incorporate the amino acid tyrosine as the 282nd amino acid in the *HFE* protein (you can confirm this for yourself by checking the genetic code table in Figure 2.2).

Figure 2.4 illustrates a portion of the *HFE* protein, which has a total of 348 amino acids in it. In Figure 2.4, the amino acids in this portion of the *HFE* protein are represented by circles. You can see the important aspects of the chemical structure of amino acid number 282 in both versions of the protein. In the version of the protein that is made by the G allele of the *HFE* gene, the 282nd amino acid in the protein is cysteine. As you can see from the figure, the amino acid cysteine has a "—CH2—SH" side group on it (the S stands for sulfur). When there is another cysteine present, the cysteines like to drop their H's and form an S—S bond between

---

[3]   The formal name for the HFE gene is the hereditary hemochromatosis gene. Please note that the abbreviations for gene names are printed in italics, while the abbreviations for protein names are printed in normal font.

[4]   Women have a lower risk for hemochromatosis than men do, because they lose iron regularly through menstruation.

[5]   The most common allele of a gene is referred to as the **wild type allele**.

them. This pulls the two cysteines toward each other, and causes the protein to bend.

Wild type HFE sequence

Nucleotide	AGA	TAT	ACG	**TGC**	CAG	GTG	GAG
Amino acid	Arg	Tyr	Thr	**Cys**	Gln	Val	Glu
	279			282			285

The G allele of the gene puts cysteine into the protein

HFE sequence with C282Y mutation

Nucleotide	AGA	TAT	ACG	**TAC**	CAG	GTG	GAG
Amino acid	Arg	Tyr	Thr	**Tyr**	Gln	Val	Glu
	279			282			285

The A allele of the gene puts tyrosine into the protein

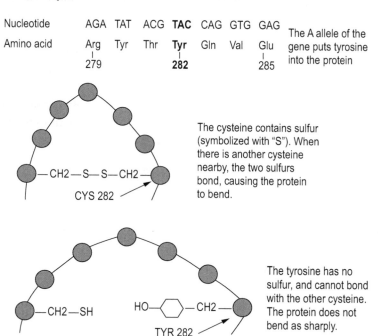

—CH2—S—S—CH2—

CYS 282

The cysteine contains sulfur (symbolized with "S"). When there is another cysteine nearby, the two sulfurs bond, causing the protein to bend.

—CH2—SH   HO—⟨ ⟩—CH2—

TYR 282

The tyrosine has no sulfur, and cannot bond with the other cysteine. The protein does not bend as sharply.

Figure 2.4 The A allele of the *HFE* gene makes a version of the *HFE* protein that does not bend properly, and therefore has reduced activity. *HFE* sequences are from the Human Genome Project, http://www.ornl.gov/sci/techresources/Human_Genome/posters/chromosome/hfe.shtml.

As Figure 2.4 illustrates, tyrosine is the 282nd amino acid in the version of the protein that is made by the A allele of the *HFE* gene[6]. As you can see from the figure, the tyrosine does not contain a sulfur atom, and therefore cannot make an S—S bond with the other cysteine. Because there is no bond between the two amino acids, this version of the HFE protein does not bend as sharply as the cysteine version does.

---

[6] Because cysteine is replaced by tyrosine as the 282nd amino acid, this mutation is referred to as a C282Y mutation. "C" and "Y" are the single-letter abbreviations for cysteine and tyrosine, respectively.

Because of the change in the protein's shape, the tyrosine version of the protein works at a lower level of activity than the cysteine version does. Because the protein works to protect you from hemochromatosis, the A allele, which produces the low-activity version of the protein, is the risk-increasing allele for this SNP. If you have the A allele for this SNP, you have a greater risk of developing hemochromatosis than you would if you had the G allele.

Special Sequences Regulate The Rate At Which The Gene Produces Its Protein

There are two ways in which a change in a gene's sequence can alter the level of activity you have of that gene's protein in your body. As described above, changes in the gene's coding sequence can cause changes in the sequence of amino acids in the protein, and that can cause changes in the level of activity of the protein. In addition, changes in certain stretches of the gene's sequence can change the rate at which the gene produces its protein, thereby causing there to be more or less of the protein in your body.

In addition to the coding sequence of the gene, each gene also has stretches of sequence where specialised proteins bind to the DNA and regulate the rate at which the gene produces its protein. These **regulatory sequences**, and the proteins that bind to them, act like the dimmer switch on a lamp. For many of your genes, the rate at which the gene produces its protein gets turned up and down as you go through your day-night cycle, your hungry-fed cycle, your menstrual cycle, and the other cycles people go through. It is well known that most genes have regulatory sequences in a region called the **promoter region** of the gene. The promoter region usually lies shortly before the beginning of the gene's coding sequence. Researchers have already discovered a number of variations in the promoter regions of genes that are believed to have medical significance. Some authorities predict that variations in regulatory sequences account for more of the person-to-person variability in risks for diseases than variations in genes' coding sequences do.

Another source of variability in the levels of activity in our proteins involves the epigenetic factors that help regulate the level of activity of some of our genes. As mentioned in chapter 1, epigenetic factors are factors that influence the rate of activity in our genes, but do not involve changes in any gene's base sequence. Your DNA gets modified chemically; one of the best-known modifications your DNA goes through involves having methyl groups (chemical formula = CH_3) put on some of the C bases in the gene's promoter region. When that happens, it can shut down that copy of the gene. As we discuss in Chapter 7, there is evidence that some of the foods and drinks we consume can affect our health by altering the epigenetic factors that regulate the activity of some of our genes.

These regulatory sequences provide a second mechanism by which person-to-person differences in a gene's sequence can result in different people having different levels of activity in that gene's protein. Even if two people have the same coding sequence of the gene, if the gene is producing its protein at different rates in the two people, the person whose gene is making more of the protein will have a higher level of that protein's activity in his/her body.

Genetic Factors Influence Your Risk For Adverse Drug Responses (ADRs) As Well

Did you know that almost half the patients who are prescribed drugs do not benefit from them? Even more alarmingly, many people experience dangerous, even potentially life-threatening side effects from their drugs; these adverse drug reactions (ADRs) account for 10-15% of emergency room admissions. Although the focus of our discussion has been on your risk for diseases, your response to prescription (and nonprescription) drugs is also a multifactorial trait. Because drugs are prescribed by doctors who practice almost every medical specialty, this is a place where personalised medicine tests can impact almost every field of medicine. If genetic tests can be developed that can predict which of several drugs and doses will be most effective for you, or reliably indicate your risk of having an ADR to the drug you are prescribed, this could save people a lot of time and money spent on ineffective treatments, and prevent a lot of the suffering that is associated with ADRs. This is an area in which there has already been some progress made, although these tests still need to be improved before they can be used for all patients.

When you take a drug, some of your proteins break the drug down chemically, and carry it out of your body. There is a large group of related proteins, called cytochrome P450 (CYP450) proteins, that metabolise a wide variety of prescription drugs. One member of the CYP450 protein family, known as CYP2D6, has a particularly variable level of activity. There are three alleles of the *CYP2D6* gene that make versions of the protein that have little to no activity. If you have one of these alleles for the *CYP2D6* gene, you will rely completely on your second copy of the *CYP2D6* gene to make enough CYP2D6 protein to metabolise the drugs that CYP2D6 metabolises. If you have two of these alleles of the *CYP2D6* gene, your body will have very little, if any, CYP2D6 protein activity. You will be classified as a "poor metaboliser" of the drugs that CYP2D6 metabolises.

Some of the people who have suffered ADRs did so because they possess two of these alleles of one of the critical *CYP450* genes, and therefore metabolised the drug so slowly that their bodies built up excessively high concentrations of the drug after a routine dose. Conversely, some of the people who have failed to improve after being given the routine dose of a commonly prescribed drug possess two high-activity alleles of a critical *CYP* gene, and metabolise the drug so quickly that their bodies never built up enough of a concentration of the drug for it to have its intended effect. At the present time, the CYP450 tests can reliably identify poor metabolisers who may have an increased risk of an ADR when they are prescribed certain drugs. These tests are not nearly as good at estimating other people's rates of drug metabolism, however, so their usefulness as a routine clinical test is limited.

CHAPTER SUMMARY

- The sequence of bases in a gene's coding sequence determines the sequence of amino acids that will be chained together to make that gene's protein. Different people often have different specific versions of the typical gene's sequence. This sometimes translates into them having different sequences of amino acids in that gene's protein.

- In order to perform its function properly, a protein must fold into a characteristic 3D shape, and be able to move to some degree as it works. The sequence of amino acids in the protein determines how comfortably the protein can fold into its characteristic shape, as well as the degree to which the protein can move. If two people have different sequences of amino acids in a protein, one version of the protein may be able to fold into its characteristic shape more comfortably than the other, or move more freely than the other. That version of the protein will have a different level of activity than the other version of the protein does.

- For most genes, different people often have slightly different versions of the gene's sequence. The difference can lie in the coding sequence of the gene, which determines the amino acids that get chained together to make the protein, or in the regulatory sequences, which control the rate at which the gene makes its protein. Some versions of the gene's sequence will cause you to have a higher or lower level of activity in that gene's protein than other versions of the gene's sequence do.

- The level of activity you have in certain proteins influences your susceptibility to many of the common multifactorial diseases, as well as how your body will respond to many drugs. Whether a particular gene allele is a risk-increasing versus risk-decreasing allele for a specific disease depends on whether that gene allele produces a version of the protein that has an unusually high or unusually low level of activity, and whether that protein creates disease-causing agents versus protects you against disease-causing agents.

CHAPTER 3

UNDERSTANDING THE PRINCIPLES OF INHERITANCE

INHERITANCE OF GENETIC FACTORS THROUGH THE GENERATIONS

In order to understand how we inherit the genetic factors that influence our risk for diseases, you need to understand a little bit about how we use chromosomes to pass our genes down to our children. Human DNA is divided into 46 separate pieces, called chromosomes. Our chromosomes are arranged in 23 pairs; the **autosomes** are referred to as chromosomes 1-22, and the **sex chromosomes** are the X and Y. Males and females both have 22 pairs of autosomes. In addition, females have two X chromosomes for their sex chromosome pair, while males have an X and a Y. Each chromosome contains a number of genes; human chromosomes range in size from the Y chromosome, which contains approximately 322 genes, to chromosome 1, which contains approximately 2,800 genes.

Each member of a chromosome pair contains the same set of genes (except X and Y). When we make sperm or eggs, we package 23 chromosomes—one from each pair—into each sperm or egg. Then, when a sperm and egg combine during fertilisation, the child ends up with the 46 chromosomes he/she needs to develop properly. This means that we possess two copies of each of our genes (except males' X and Y genes), but we only pass down one copy of each of our genes to each of our children.

Figures 3.1 and 3.2 illustrate the basic principles of gene alleles and inheritance. Recall from Chapter 2 that there are many different specific versions, or alleles, of any given gene. Figure 3.1 illustrates one possible set of allele combinations for two genes that somebody's father and mother might have. In this figure, Gene 1 lies on chromosome 1, while Gene 2 lies on chromosome 2. The pair of alleles a person has for a particular gene is referred to as that person's **genotype** for that gene. Both Gene 1 and Gene 2 have SNPs in their coding sequences. Let's say that, if you looked at these SNPs in a large number of people, you would find all four possible alleles of both these SNPs in the population. Some people would have an A nucleotide in that position (i.e. they would have the A allele), some would have a C nucleotide in that position (the C allele), some would have a G nucleotide (the G allele), and still others would have a T nucleotide (the T allele). In these particular individuals, however, the father has the GT genotype (he possesses both the G and T alleles) for Gene 1, while the mother has the

CG genotype (she possesses both the C and G alleles). Because they have two different alleles for this gene, the father and mother are said to be **heterozygous** for this gene's alleles. For Gene 2, on the other hand, the father has the AG genotype, while the mother has the TT genotype. The mother is said to be **homozygous** for the alleles of this gene, because she has two copies of the same T allele.

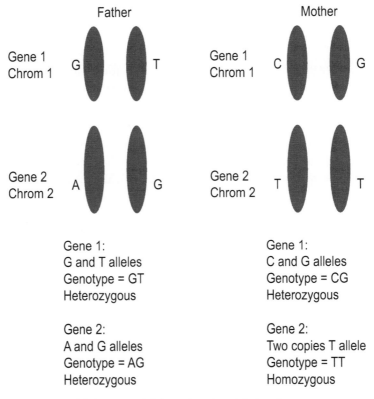

Figure 3.1 One possible set of alleles someone's father and mother might have for two genes.

Figure 3.2 illustrates the allele combinations for Gene 1 that a child of this couple could possibly inherit. Because he has the GT genotype, the father could package either the G allele or the T allele into any given sperm. Because she has the CG genotype, the mother could package either the C allele or the G allele into any given egg. This means that, for Gene 1, there are four possible genotypes a child could inherit: CG, GG, CT or GT. The alleles that the child inherits for Gene 1 will be one of the genetic factors that influence the child's susceptibility to the diseases or drug reactions that are influenced by the function of Gene 1's protein. If the child's alleles produce versions of their proteins that have significantly higher or lower levels of activity than the typical person's versions do, the child will be either more or less susceptible to certain diseases or drug reactions than the typical person is.

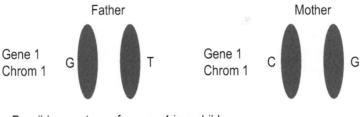

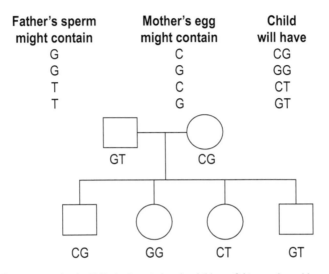

Figure 3.2 The genotypes for the SNPs in Gene 1 that the children of this couple could possibly inherit.

SINGLE-GENE DISEASES PRODUCE MENDELIAN PATTERNS OF INHERITANCE

Gregor Mendel Described The Inheritance Of Single-Gene Traits

You may have heard the terms "dominant" and "recessive" used to describe disease-causing gene mutations or genetic diseases. These terms refer to some of the basic rules of inheritance that Gregor Mendel first laid down when he did his pioneering work in genetics. Gregor Mendel (1822-1884) was a monk who studied the inheritance of traits in pea plants, and established the basic rules of inheritance. It is interesting to note, however, that the rules of inheritance that Mendel laid down only apply to traits (and diseases) that are controlled by a single gene. Mendel began studying approximately 20 traits in his pea plants, but ended up only studying about seven traits. Each of these traits is controlled by a single gene, and therefore is inherited in a predictable pattern. Mendel could not establish a predictable pattern of inheritance for the other thirteen traits, which were multifactorial traits, so he focused on the traits for which he could see a predictable pattern of inheritance in each new generation.

Single-gene traits are the only kind of trait Mendel could have studied in order to discover the basic rules of inheritance, because they are the only traits that are inherited in predictable patterns. If one parent has a particular single-gene trait, you can usually predict what the probability is that any of that parent's offspring will also have that trait. Because multifactorial traits are influenced not only by multiple genetic factors that are inherited, but also by nongenetic factors that are not inherited, it is considerably harder to predict the probability that a parent with a given multifactorial trait will produce a child with the same trait.

There are over 6,000 single-gene diseases that have been described; a few are listed in Table 3-1. These diseases account for approximately 4% of all people with significant disease in the general population. The laws of inheritance that Mendel passed down apply well to single-gene diseases. They enable genetic counselors to provide people who possess disease-causing gene mutations with accurate estimates of the risk they will have an affected child, or the probability that a family member also has that mutation. There are several different types of single-gene, or Mendelian, patterns of inheritance that you can see in families that possess disease-causing gene mutations.

Autosomal Dominant Inheritance

The term "autosomal dominant" refers to a situation in which the gene mutation that is causing the disease is on one of the numbered chromosomes (autosomes), and only one of your two copies of the gene needs to have the mutation in order for you to develop the disease (because the mutation will dominate over the good copy of the gene). In a family with an autosomal dominant mutation, the disease will not skip a generation. An affected person will have inherited the disease-causing mutation from one of his/her parents, who would be affected him/herself[1]. He/she will also have a 50% chance of passing the mutation down to each of his/her children, so you expect approximately

---

[1] The exception to this is the first person in the family to have the disease. Neither this person's mother nor his/her father possessed the mutation. The mutation arose as either the egg or sperm that created him/her was made.

half his/her children to be affected also[2]. An unaffected person does not possess the mutation; his/her children will all be unaffected.

Table 3-1. Some Single-Gene Diseases

Disease	Symptoms
Autosomal Recessive	
Cystic fibrosis	Chronic lung infections and congestion, poor weight gain, salty sweat, male infertility
Spinal muscular atrophy	Various forms cause progressive muscle degeneration and weakness
Hemochromatosis	Organs in the body retain excessive iron, leading to high risk for infection; damage to the heart, liver and pancreas; abnormal skin pigmentation
Sickle cell disease	Anemia, spleen damage, joint pain, high risk of infection
Autosomal Dominant	
Achondroplasia	The most common form of dwarfism, with short limbs, and normal size head and trunk
Familial hypercholesterolemia	Very high level of cholesterol in the blood; high risk for heart disease
Huntington disease	Progressive loss of motor control and personality change beginning in middle age
Lactose intolerance	Inability to digest lactose (milk sugar), causing cramps, bloating and flatulence after eating dairy foods
Polycystic kidney disease (one form)	Development of cysts in the kidney, causing blood in the urine, high blood pressure, abdominal pain

An autosomal dominant disease can be passed down through either the mother or the father, and sons and daughters are equally likely to be affected with the disease. Figure 3.3 depicts a pedigree that illustrates autosomal dominant inheritance. In Chapter 4 we will discuss how pedigrees are constructed in more detail. For now, it is important to know that in pedigree illustrations, female family members are drawn as circles, while male family members are drawn as squares. If a person has a disease (especially in the case of single gene disease), the symbol is shaded in. As we discuss below, it is also

---

[2]   This assumes that the affected person only has one mutant copy of the gene. This will usually be the case. It is possible for someone to have a dominant mutation in both copies of the gene, but if having that dominant mutation in one copy of the gene is enough to cause a disease, having that mutation in both copies of the gene is often lethal, or will at least render that person unable to reproduce.

possible for someone to have a recessive mutation in one copy of the gene, but not be affected by the disease. These people's symbols are not shaded in, but they have dots in the middle of them.

In this family, the paternal grandfather (I-1) of the proband[3] (III-2, indicated by an arrow) has the mutation, and is affected by the disease. His son II-2 and daughter II-3 have both inherited the mutation from him, and both also have the disease. His son II-4 and daughter II-5, on the other hand, have not inherited the mutation, and do not have the disease. II-2 has passed the mutation down to his daughter III-2, who has the disease.

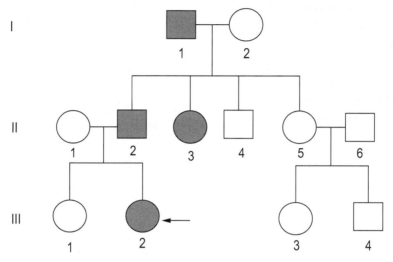

Figure 3.3 Pedigree illustrating autosomal dominant inheritance

Autosomal Recessive Inheritance

The term "autosomal recessive" refers to a situation in which the mutant gene is on one of the numbered chromosomes (autosomes), and you must have a mutation in both copies of the gene in order for you to develop the disease (because the mutation will be recessive to a normal copy of the gene). In a family with an autosomal recessive mutation, the disease may skip one or more generations. People who only have the mutation in one copy of the gene are unaffected carriers of the mutation. Even though they do not have the disease, they still have the mutation, and therefore have a 50% chance of passing the mutation down to any given child. A family can have many members who are unaffected carriers of the mutation. However, in order to be affected, a child must inherit the mutation from both parents, which means that both parents must be unaffected carriers of the mutation.

---

3   The proband is the first person in the family to have brought the family to the attention of health care providers.

It is estimated that the typical person carries 50-100 recessive mutations. Fortunately, however, unrelated people usually have their recessive mutations in different genes. In this case, even if a child inherits all his/her parents' recessive mutations, he/she won't have a mutation in both copies of any given gene, and therefore he/she will not have a disease. The more closely two people are related, however, the more likely they are to have recessive mutations in the same gene. If both parents carry an autosomal recessive mutation in the same gene, each parent has a 50% chance of passing the mutation down to a child, and the child has a 25% chance of developing the associated recessive disease.

Figure 3.4 depicts a pedigree that illustrates autosomal recessive inheritance. I-2 has the mutation in both copies of the gene, and therefore has the disease. Because her husband I-1 does not have the mutation, however, none of their children has the disease. Their son II-2 and their daughter II-5 are unaffected carriers of the mutation. Because II-2 married a woman who also carries the mutation, they have the ability to produce an affected child. Their son III-4 (the proband in this pedigree) has inherited the mutation from both his parents, and therefore has the disease.

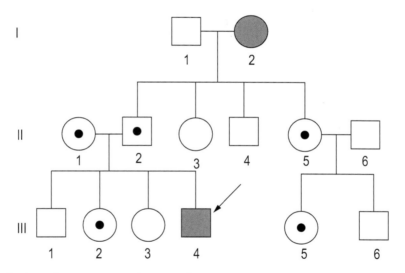

Figure 3.4 Pedigree illustrating autosomal recessive inheritance

X-Linked Recessive Inheritance

The term "X-linked" refers to a situation in which the gene that has the mutation lies on the X chromosome. In a family with an X-linked recessive mutation, many more males are affected than females. If a daughter inherits a mutation, she has a good copy of the gene to compensate for the mutation. Males, on the other hand, only have one copy of their X chromosome genes, so if a son inherits a mutation, he will have the disease. Because a son gets his X chromosome from his mother, all males who have an X-linked recessive disease inherited their mutations from their mothers. Because his only copy of that X-linked gene has a mutation in it, an affected male will pass the mutation down to all his daughters.

Figure 3.5 depicts a pedigree that illustrates X-linked recessive inheritance. I-2 has passed her mutation down to her son II-2 and her daughter II-4. Because her son II-2 does not have a good copy of the gene to compensate for the copy with the mutation, he has the disease. Because her daughter II-4 inherited a normal copy of the gene from her father, she is an unaffected carrier of the mutation.

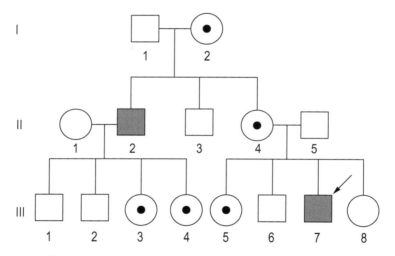

Figure 3.5 Pedigree illustrating X-linked recessive inheritance

X-linked Dominant Inheritance

As is true for X-linked recessive mutations, if a male inherits an X-linked dominant mutation, he will be affected. In addition, a female who inherits an X-linked dominant mutation will also be affected, even if the other copy of that gene is normal. In a family with an X-linked dominant mutation, every affected male has an affected mother[4]. In addition, approximately half an affected woman's children will inherit her mutation

---

[4]   Except for the occasional situation in which the first person affected in the family was a male whose mutation arose as his mother was making the egg that created him.

as well[5]. Because he only has one copy of his X chromosome genes, an affected male will pass the mutation down to each of his daughters, who will be affected. None of his sons will inherit the mutation, however, because they will inherit their father's Y chromosome, not his X.

Figure 3.6 depicts a pedigree that illustrates X-linked dominant inheritance. I-2 has a mutation in one copy of the gene in question, and consequently has the disease. Her son II-2 and her daughter II-4 have both inherited the mutation, and both of them have the disease as well. Because II-2 only has one X chromosome, and a man passes his X chromosome to his daughters, both of II-2's daughters (III-3 and III-4) have inherited the mutation. Neither of his sons have, however, because a son inherits his father's Y chromosome, not his X. Because II-4 has inherited a normal copy of the gene from her father (you know I-1's copy is normal, because if he had the mutation he would have the disease), she can pass down either the normal copy or the copy with the mutation in it to her children.

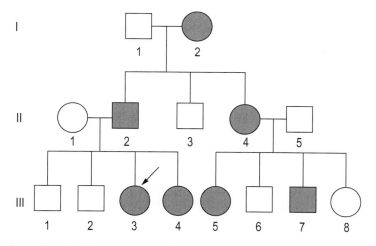

Figure 3.6 Pedigree illustrating X-linked dominant inheritance

Some Women May Be More Or Less Severely Affected By An X-Linked Mutation Than You Would Predict

In most cases, you can predict how severely a woman will be affected by an X-linked mutation by determining whether the mutation is dominant or recessive, and determining how many copies of the gene in question have the mutation. In some cases, however, there is another factor that can influence how severely the woman is affected by

---

[5] This assumes the affected woman only has one mutant copy of the gene. This is usually true. A woman who has two X-linked dominant mutations in the same gene will probably be too severely affected to reproduce.

the mutation she has. In every woman's cells, one of her two X chromosomes is inactivated. Most, but not all, of the genes on the inactive X chromosome are turned off permanently. It appears that it is best to have only one working copy of many of the genes that lie on the X chromosome, whether you are a man or a woman. It also appears, however, that there are some X chromosome genes for which a woman needs to have two working copies.

This means that, with respect to the effects of her X-linked gene mutation on her health, a woman's body contains two populations of cells: cells that have inactivated the X chromosome she inherited from her father and cells that have inactivated the X chromosome she inherited from her mother. The cells that inactivate the X chromosome that carries the gene mutation will be saved from any negative effects the mutation would have on the cells' health. The cells that leave the mutation-bearing X chromosome active, however, will suffer from the negative effects the mutation has on the cells' health. In most women, there are approximately equal numbers of cells in the two populations (this is referred to as having **balanced X inactivation**). Cells from both populations live side-by-side in each of her tissues and organs. In approximately 10% of women, however, there are a lot more cells that belong to one population than the other (referred to as **skewed X inactivation**).

We expect a woman to be affected by an X-linked dominant mutation, but not affected if only one copy of the relevant gene has an X-linked recessive mutation. This is based on the expectation that her X inactivation will be balanced, however. Figure 3.7 illustrates the way in which skewed X inactivation can cause the woman to be either more severely or less severely affected by the mutation than you would expect. In Figure 3.7, the woman has inherited an X-linked mutation from her mother, and a normal copy of the gene from her father. In the top portion of the figure, the mutation is an X-linked recessive mutation. If her X inactivation is balanced, we expect her to be healthy. If, however, 95% of her cells inactivate the X chromosome she inherited from her father, then those cells will all suffer from the effects of the mutation, and she will be more affected than you would expect her to be. In the bottom portion of the figure, the mutation is an X-linked dominant mutation. If the woman's X inactivation is balanced, we expect her to have the disease. However, if 95% of her cells have inactivated the X chromosome she inherited from her mother, only 5% of her cells will suffer from the effects of the mutation, and she will be less affected than you would expect her to be.

Y-Linked Inheritance

There are not very many Y-linked traits; it appears that the Y chromosome does not have very many genes on it. A disease that was due to a mutation on a Y chromosome gene would be passed from an affected male to all his sons. Females would never develop the disease, because they don't have a Y chromosome.

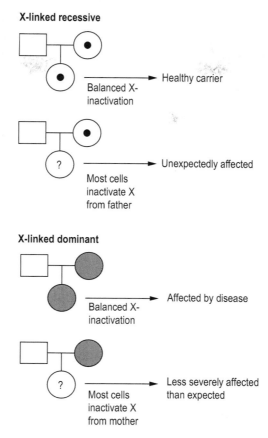

Figure 3.7 Skewed X inactivation can cause a woman to be more or less affected by an X-linked gene mutation than one would expect.

THE PATTERNS OF INHERITANCE SEEN WITH MULTIFACTORIAL DISEASES ARE LESS PREDICTABLE (AT THE PRESENT TIME) THAN THOSE SEEN WITH SINGLE-GENE DISORDERS

Many Genetic And Nongenetic Factors Are As Yet Undiscovered

In contrast to the predictable patterns of inheritance and risk for family members that you see in families that have single-gene disorders, the pattern of inheritance and risk for individual family members you see with most multifactorial disorders is much less predictable. There are several reasons why this is true. One is that we do not yet know what all of the critical genetic and nongenetic factors are for most multifactorial diseases (like most forms of cancer, or heart disease). For example, researchers are just beginning to discover the role that somatic mutations and mitochondrial DNA mutations (discussed in the next section) play in influencing your risk for diseases. Another is the fact that many of these multifactorial diseases do not develop until late in life. This may make it hard to gauge your risk by studying your family history. Some members of your family who are disease-free at the time you collected your family history data will actually develop the disease later on. The fact that they were disease-free when you collected their information may cause you to underestimate the number of family members you have with the disease, and underestimate your own risk for the disease as well.

Once researchers discover what the critical genetic and nongenetic factors are that influence a particular disease, and the complex way in which they interact, they can assemble them into a formula that can predict your risk for the disease accurately. One of the most important goals of personalised medicine research is to determine what the critical genetic and nongenetic factors are for the different multifactorial diseases, and how to assemble them into formulas that accurately predict your risk of developing each specific disease.

Somatic Mutations And Mitochondrial Mutations Also Contribute To Multifactorial Diseases

The discussion so far has focused on the genes that are on your chromosomes, and the means by which they are passed down from your parents. In order to include all the ways in which your DNA affects your health, however, there are two other types of gene mutations we need to consider: **somatic mutations** and **mitochondrial DNA mutations**. Mitochondrial DNA mutations can be inherited or acquired, while somatic mutations are acquired, typically by exposure to things in our environment that damages our DNA.

As Figure 3.8 illustrates, we begin life as a fertilised egg. From there we need to not only produce approximately 100 trillion cells to make a human body, but we also need to develop approximately 210 different types of tissues, each one made of cells that have their own unique structural and functional characteristics. For example, some cells need to become bone cells, while others need to become muscle cells. Still others need to become skin cells, while others need to become the cells that line your eyeballs. Each type of tissue has a very different set of physical and functional characteristics.

In order to make the trillions of cells that are required to make a human body, our cells undergo repeated rounds of **replication and division**. The cell first makes a copy of everything it has inside it (to replicate = to copy), including the DNA, then splits (division) into two daughter cells. With 3.3 billion nucleotides in your DNA, every time a cell replicates its DNA, there is a chance that a mutation can arise in one of its genes. If a mutation does arise, when the cell divides, one of its two daughter cells will receive the gene with the mutation in it. As that daughter cell continues to replicate and divide, the mutation will be present in the cells that descend from the cell in which the mutation originally appeared.

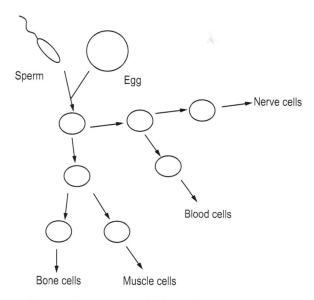

Figure 3.8 In order to make the number and variety of cells your body needs, your cells undergo repeated cycles of replication, division and differentiation into different cell types.

These kinds of mutations are called somatic mutations (from the Latin soma = body). There are several important differences between somatic mutations and **germline mutations**, which are mutations that are present in the sperm or egg that created you. Somatic mutations are often caused by things we encounter through our diet, environment or lifestyle. They are not inherited, but rather acquired over the course of our lifetime. In addition, germline mutations are present in every cell of your body. In contrast, somatic mutations are only present in a subset of your cells. Somatic mutations can cause the cells that have them to function abnormally, however, and if you accumulate enough somatic mutations, you may develop a multifactorial disease.

Somatic mutations play an important role in the development of several diseases, but they are best known for their ability to contribute to several types of cancers. Each of your cells has a certain lifespan, just as you do yourself. Each cell is supposed to undergo a certain number of cycles of replication and division, then die. For example, the cells that make up the lining of the colon should turn over every 7-10 days. There are over

100 different specific types of cancer. Every cancer, no matter what specific type, begins when a single cell continues to replicate and divide after it is supposed to have died. Normally, before any cell can undergo another cycle of replication and division, there are a number of proteins that check several aspects of the cell's age and health, and certify that the cell is young enough and healthy enough to undergo another cycle of replication and division. If this cell cycle control system fails to function properly, the cell continues to replicate and divide, even after it has reached what was supposed to be the end of its lifespan.

Figure 3.9 illustrates how colorectal cancer develops from the accumulation of several gene mutations. Although a small percentage of cancers involve germline mutations in the relevant genes, the vast majority (80-90%) involve somatic mutations that accumulate in cells that were genetically normal when they were first produced. In the case of colon cancer, the colorectal tumor progresses in several stages, and each step is marked by a different type of genetic change.

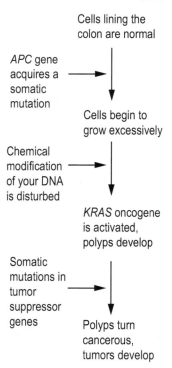

Colorectal cancer can develop as a result of accumulated mutations

Cells lining the colon are normal

APC gene acquires a somatic mutation

Cells begin to grow excessively

Chemical modification of your DNA is disturbed

KRAS oncogene is activated, polyps develop

Somatic mutations in tumor suppressor genes

Polyps turn cancerous, tumors develop

Figure 3.9 A colorectal tumor develops in stages, each of which is accompanied by a change in the activity of certain genes.

Two types of genes are involved: **oncogenes** and **tumor suppressor genes**. Oncogenes are genes that promote cell replication and division. While we need them to be active during the early stages of our lives, when we need to make many new cells to create the tissues and organs our bodies need, at some point we need them to be turned off in most of our cells. If an oncogene that has been turned off because your body no longer needs it to be active is reactivated in a population of cells, those cells will grow excessively, and cancer may result. Tumor suppressor genes make proteins that cause cells that are trying to grow out of control to die. Losing the function of tumor suppressor genes can allow these tumors to grow.

In this scenario, a somatic mutation in a gene called *APC* causes one of the cells that line the colon to begin to replicate and divide excessively. This creates a population of cells lining the colon that are growing out of control. Chemical modifications of your DNA (discussed in Chapter 7) regulate the activity of many of your genes. In this case, the *KRAS* oncogene, which has been turned off at this point, is reactivated because the chemical modifications that caused it to be silenced are reversed. Once *KRAS* is reactivated, the cells that are now growing out of control form a polyp. If one or more additional tumor suppressor or oncogenes in the polyp cells acquires additional somatic mutations, a colorectal tumor develops.

The other type of DNA we need to consider is **mitochondrial DNA**. The **mitochondrion** is an **organelle** (the cell's version of an organ) that functions as the cell's energy generator. The mitochondrion is the place where we harvest most of the energy we get from our food. In addition to that very important function, however, the mitochondrion also has its own DNA molecule, which contains 37 genes, each of which makes a protein that is essential to your health.

Mitochondrial DNA mutations can be either inherited or acquired after birth. We inherit all our mitochondria from our mothers, so we will inherit any mitochondrial DNA mutations our mother has. In addition, mitochondrial DNA mutates at a higher rate than the DNA in our chromosomes does, and has less ability to repair mutations that do arise. This means that as we age, we accumulate mutations in our mitochondrial DNA. Fortunately, we have a huge number of mitochondrial DNA molecules in our bodies. Each cell has multiple mitochondria in it (sometimes hundreds), and each mitochondrion has multiple copies (up to a dozen or so) of the mitochondrial DNA molecule in it. Therefore, many cells have hundreds, even thousands, of copies of the mitochondrial DNA molecule in them. This allows us to hold out for a long time against the rising number of mitochondrial DNA mutations. If a particular population of cells accumulate enough mitochondrial gene mutations, however, this can increase our risk for certain multifactorial diseases.

A Note About Inheritance When There Are Multiple Children In the Family

When you are trying to calculate the probability that a parent with a gene mutation (for single-gene diseases) or a risk-increasing allele (for multifactorial diseases) may pass that allele down to his/her children, you need to avoid committing what is known as the "gambler's fallacy." There are two versions of the gambler's fallacy. You can think that, because something has not happened recently, it is more likely to happen than it actually is. Alternatively, you can think that, because something has happened recently, it is less likely to happen again than it actually is. For example, if you are rolling two six-sided dice, the probability of rolling a double 4 on any single roll is 1 in 36. If you roll the dice 1,000 times and a double 4 does not come up, the probability of rolling a double 4 on the next roll is still 1 in 36. Similarly, if you roll a double 4, the probability of rolling a second double 4 on the very next roll is 1 in 36. Whether you have rolled a double 4 recently or not, the probability of rolling a double 4 on any given roll is 1 in 36.

This same principle also applies to your children's probabilities of inheriting any disease-causing mutations (for single-gene diseases) or risk-increasing alleles (for multifactorial diseases) you possess. Imagine, for example, that you have an autosomal dominant mutation that causes a single-gene disease, and your second copy of that gene has a normal sequence. Your probability of passing the mutation down to a child is 50%. If you pass that mutation down to your first child, the probability that you will pass the mutation down to the next child is also 50%. Because each child is created from a different egg and a different sperm, the fact that the first child inherited the mutation does not change the probability that the second child will inherit it. Similarly, if you have three unaffected children, who did not inherit the mutation, the probability your fourth child will inherit the mutation is still 50%.

Chapter Summary

- Your mother and father each have two copies of each of their genes (except for your father having one copy of his X and Y chromosome genes). You inherited one of the two copies of each gene that your father possesses, and one copy of each of the genes your mother possesses.

- Single-gene diseases often exhibit predictable patterns of inheritance, ex. autosomal dominant, autosomal recessive, X-linked recessive, X-linked dominant or Y-linked.

- The patterns of inheritance seen for multifactorial diseases are not as predictable as those seen for single-gene diseases, because we have not yet discovered many of the critical genetic and nongenetic factors that contribute to multifactorial diseases, and do not understand all the complex ways in which they interact with each other.

- Somatic mutations arise after fertilisation of the egg, during a time when your cells are repeatedly undergoing cycles of replication and division. They only appear in a subset of your cells. They can contribute to multifactorial diseases, however, because they can impair the function of those cells. They are especially important contributors to cancer.

- Your mitochondria are better known as the energy provider for your cells, but they also have their own DNA, which contains 37 genes, each of which makes a protein that is essential for your health. Mutations in mitochondrial genes can also contribute to multifactorial diseases, because they can impair your cells' ability to function, or to withstand the impact of nongenetic factors on their function.

- When you are calculating the probability that someone's children will inherit a mutation, risk-increasing allele or disease, you must consider each child a separate, independent case. Whether previous children have inherited the mutation or allele does not change the probability that future children will inherit it.

CHAPTER 4

USING YOUR FAMILY HISTORY INFORMATION TO PREDICT YOUR RISK FOR SPECIFIC DISEASES

YOUR FAMILY HISTORY MAY PROVIDE MORE INFORMATION THAN YOU THINK

Although genetic and genomic testing will soon become an important tool to help you learn more about your risk for disease and what you can do to improve your health, we are only beginning to understand how to make sense of the enormous amount of information that is generated from these powerful new technologies. One thing you should keep in mind, however, is that you have a valuable tool that is already available to you, that provides information that is fairly easy to understand, and that can tell you quite a lot about your risk for certain diseases. This tool is your family medical history. Whether you are considering single-gene diseases such as cystic fibrosis or multifactorial diseases such as diabetes or heart disease, your family history can help you learn more about your risk. In fact, even in this new era of whole-genome sequencing and genome-wide association studies, your family history remains the single least expensive and most effective means by which you can estimate your risk for the disorders for which you have the greatest genetic risk.

In order for you to be sure you include all the relevant information in your family history, you should include not only the diseases that have affected your family members, but also as much information as you can about your relatives' dietary, environmental, lifestyle, behavioral and cultural factors. These nongenetic factors can strongly influence your risk for some multifactorial diseases, and may even affect the way some single-gene disorders affect people. It is also important to know your specific ethnic and religious heritage on both your mother's and your father's side of the family. Ethnicity and religious heritage can, at times, indicate additional risk for certain genetic diseases, such as hereditary forms of breast cancer in people of Eastern European Ashkenazi Jewish descent.

Your family history may actually serve two very important purposes. First, it can help inform you about your level of risk for certain diseases. Second, it can help you identify things you can change about your diet, environment and lifestyle to reduce your overall risk of developing the diseases for which you have the most genetic risk. Recall that one of the most important principles of personalised medicine is that, if you know which diseases you have the greatest genetic risk for, which is something you cannot control, you may be able to adjust your diet, environment and lifestyle to reduce your exposure to the nongenetic risk factors that you can control.

Knowing your family history can literally can be a lifesaver. By noticing patterns of disease within your family, you and your healthcare team may be able to determine that you have an increased risk for a disease even before you exhibit symptoms. This may help your health care team design a program of screening, management and/or dietary, environmental and lifestyle changes that will reduce your overall risk of developing the disease. Given the dynamic nature of any family history, the family medical history should be reviewed and updated on a regular basis.

DRAWING YOUR FAMILY TREE

Figure 4.1 illustrates the common symbols used to draw pedigrees (the formal name for family trees). Squares are used to indicate males, circles are used to indicate females, and diamonds are used when an individual's (often a fetus) sex is not known. The person who first brings the family to medical attention is known as the **proband**, and is indicated by an arrow. As is indicated in the third line of the figure, mating is indicated by a single horizontal line between a male and a female, unless the two are related, in which case a double horizontal line is used.

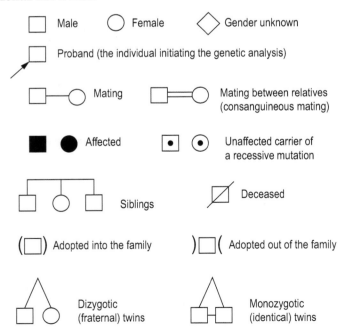

Figure 4.1 The symbols that are commonly used to draw human pedigrees.

Healthy family members are indicated by unfilled symbols. Affected individuals' (people that have a particular disease, like cancer) symbols are filled in; filling in the affected people's symbols allows you to more clearly see the pattern of inheritance of the disease. When someone has a recessive mutation in only one of his/her two copies of a particular gene, that individual's symbol will have a dot in the middle of it (sometimes the symbol will be half filled in). As we discussed in Chapter 3, if a mutation is recessive, both copies of that gene must have the mutation in order for the individual to be affected. Consequently, people who only have one mutant copy of the gene are expected to be unaffected if the mutation is recessive.

A set of siblings (brothers and sisters) is indicated by the appropriate number of squares and circles hanging down from a horizontal line. Twins descend on diagonal lines from the same point; monozygotic (identical) twins have a horizontal line drawn between them. Family members who are deceased are usually indicated by a diagonal line running through their symbols. Family members who were adopted into the family have their symbols enclosed in inward-facing brackets, while family members who were adopted out of the family have their symbols enclosed in outward-facing brackets.

Figure 4.2 illustrates a hypothetical family pedigree, and specifies each family member's relationship to you.

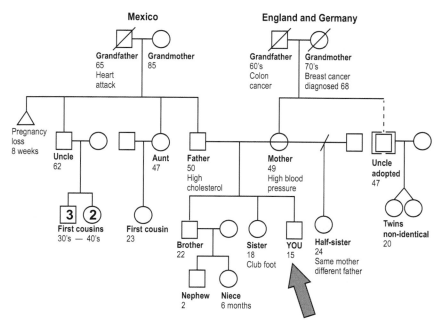

Figure 4.2 A hypothetical human pedigree, or family tree. The different family members' relationships to you (indicated by an arrow) are indicated. From http://www.geneticalliance.org/ksc_assets/pdfs/manual/chapter_3.pdf

My Family Health Portrait: An Internet Program You Can Access To Draw Your Family's Pedigree And Summarise The Relevant Information From Your Family History

There is often valuable information to be gotten from studying a person's family history. Unfortunately, however, few people appreciate how useful family history information can be. In addition, the average duration of an encounter between a patient and his/her primary-care physician is far too short to enable the doctor to gather all the pertinent family information.

On November 8, 2004, Surgeon General Richard H. Carmona launched a national initiative to encourage people to learn more about their family medical history. Thanksgiving Day was declared National Family History Day, and it was emphasised that family gatherings such as Thanksgiving celebrations, family reunions and weddings provide excellent opportunities to gather and update family history information.

The Surgeon General's office maintains a website (https://familyhistory.hhs.gov/fhh-web/home.action) called My Family Health Portrait, which enables you to generate a printable family pedigree. You can download the tool to a home computer, for control and privacy. Drawing your family tree using this tool allows you to easily update or change the information at a later time. Because the information is in electronic form, you can share it with your family members and your healthcare team. Because the tool is based on commonly used standards for electronic health records, it may be possible to have this information go directly into your electronic health record. At this time, this tool does not help you estimate your risk for any of the diseases that appear in your family, but it does enable you to generate a printed family pedigree with everyone's health history and relevant nongenetic factors on it. This way, you can arrive for your doctor's appointment with all the relevant information organised in a manner that enables the doctor to search quickly for information that can guide decisions about your health care.

This website is free to the public, and very easy to use. It asks you how many of each type of relative you have, whether any of your relatives are twins or adopted, and draws a pedigree that represents your family. The site allows you to indicate on the pedigree any diseases that affect(ed) your family members. In addition, to provide your doctor with all the relevant information, add any information you can remember about each individual's occupation, as well as any other dietary, environmental or lifestyle factors you can think of that might have exposed that person to a disease-causing agent. You can then share this with your doctor, who can carefully consider the relevant aspects of your family's medical history as he/she estimates your genetic risk for the diseases that have appeared in your family. In many cases, contacting a genetic counselor can also help you better understand your disease risk based on family medical history.

Even If You Have A Family Member With A Disease, This Does Not Necessarily Put You At High Risk

Even if you have a family member with one of the common multifactorial diseases, this does not necessarily mean that you have a high risk for contracting that disease yourself. In fact, if you have a fairly large family, and have just one first degree relative (parent, sibling or child) with a multifactorial disease, your chances of developing that disease yourself are only 3-15%, depending on the specific disease. If you have a small family, it may be harder to use your family history to estimate your risk, especially for diseases that affect one sex more often or more severely than the other.

There are several reasons why you might not develop the disease that affected some of your relatives. In fact, there are several reasons why you might not even have a heavy genetic load for that disease, even if you have family members who are affected with the disease. To begin with, if nongenetic factors contributed to your relatives' disease more strongly than genetic factors did, there may be few genetic factors for you to worry about inheriting. Further, if you can identify the nongenetic factors that contributed to the disease in your relative, you may be able to avoid them, and thereby avoid developing the disease.

If members of more than one generation share the critical nongenetic factors, a disease that is largely due to nongenetic factors can produce a pattern of disease in the family that resembles the pattern of inheritance you sometimes get when the disease is due solely to a genetic factor. For example, one of us authors (RCM) has a strong family history of skin cancer. My parents have always loved the beach and boating, as has my paternal grandfather (my father's father). When I was young, the health experts of the time claimed that you should soak up as much sun as possible, because it was good for your health in many ways. Nowadays, we understand that excessive sun exposure is an important risk factor for skin cancer, and that, if you were exposed to excessive sunlight when you were a child, you have a high risk for skin cancer, no matter how careful you have been to avoid overexposure in recent years.

My father has had a cancerous growth surgically removed from his head, as did his father before him. There are three main types of skin cancers: melanoma, basal cell carcinoma and squamous cell carcinoma. Some forms of melanoma are caused largely by genetic factors, but the squamous form of skin cancer, which is the type that was found in my father and grandfather, is considered to be caused primarily by nongenetic factors such as excessive sun exposure. Both my father and grandfather were avid fishermen, as well as beach-goers and boaters, and spent a great deal of time in the sun. Because excessive sun exposure is such an important risk factor for this type of cancer, I wear hats and use sunscreen when I go out in the sun. In addition, because I understand that the precautions I currently take may not be enough to prevent a cancer from developing, I have a dermatologist examine me for possible skin cancers every year.

Even if one of your parents carries a significant genetic load, such as for a single gene disease, you may not have inherited the genetic factors that predisposed him/her to the disease. Remember that we each have two copies, or alleles, of each of our genes[1], and we pass one of those two alleles down to each child. Even if your parent had one risk-increasing allele for several critical genes, you may have inherited the other alleles of those genes, and have a typical level of risk for that disease.

Another reason why having an affected relative does not necessarily mean you will have a high genetic risk for that disease involves the fact that not all the genetic factors that can contribute to multifactorial diseases can be inherited by the affected person's children. As we discussed in Chapter 3, a somatic mutation arises after fertilisation, while the embryo's cells are replicating and dividing. A somatic mutation only appears in a subset of the individual's cells—cells that descended from the cell in which the mutation originally arose.

If the somatic mutation is present only in the lung cells, or cells in the liver, it can contribute to that person having a multifactorial disease, because the organ whose cells contain the mutation will not function properly. It will not get passed down to any of the individual's children, however, because a mutation that exists only in the lung cells or liver cells cannot get packaged into the sperm or eggs that individual makes. In some cases, however, the cells in the testes that make sperm, or the cells in the ovaries that make eggs will have the somatic mutation in them. In these cases, some of the sperm or eggs that individual makes will have the mutation in them, and any child that results from the fertilisation of a mutation-bearing sperm or egg will have the mutation in all his/her cells. In most cases, however, the somatic mutations a parent possesses will not be present in the testes or ovaries. Therefore, if one of your parents had a multifactorial disease, and somatic mutations were an important factor causing it, you are probably not going to inherit these mutations.

Recall also that the mitochondria, better known for supplying the cells with chemical energy, also have their own DNA, and that the proteins that the mitochondrial genes make are also critical to your health. During fertilisation, the sperm donates its DNA to the new child, and very little else. All the mitochondria the embryo will rely on to provide energy for its cells come from the egg. Consequently, we get all our mitochondria from our mother. A woman with a mitochondrial gene mutation will pass the mutation to all her children, sons and daughters alike. If your father had a multifactorial disease, however, and an accumulation of mitochondrial gene mutations was partly responsible

---

[1]   Except for males having one copy of their X and Y chromosome genes, and everyone having many copies of their mitochondrial DNA genes.

for it, you would not inherit any of the mitochondrial gene mutations that contributed to your father's disease.

Figure 4.3 illustrates some of the possible reasons why your risk for a particular multifactorial disease may be relatively low, even if one of your parents has the disease.

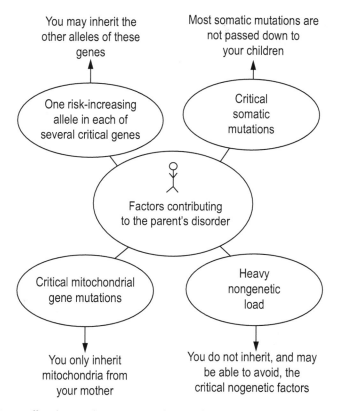

Figure 4.3 Having an affected parent does not necessarily mean that you have inherited a heavy genetic load for that particular disease.

THE NUMBER OF AFFECTED RELATIVES, HOW CLOSE THEY ARE TO YOU, AND AT WHAT AGE THEY WERE AFFECTED ARE ALL RELEVANT

Your family history can often provide you, your doctor or your genetic counselor with important information that can help you estimate your risk for the disease(s) that have appeared in your family. It is important to understand, however, exactly how the number of affected relatives you have, how closely related they are to you and the age at which they were diagnosed with the disease influence your genetic risk, to insure that you end up with the most accurate possible estimate of your risk.

As you probably already understand, the more affected relatives you have with a particular disease, the more likely it is that genetic factors are making a strong contribution to the disease in your family. If you have a number of relatives affected with a particular disease, however, before you conclude that your family has one or more risk-increasing genetic factors running through it, you need to be sure that the affected individuals didn't all share some dietary, environmental or lifestyle factor that could have had a strong influence on their susceptibility to that disease. For example, growing up in a family of cigarette smokers will increase your risk not only for lung cancer but also other respiratory system diseases. When you draw up your family's pedigree, it is important to include information about each individual's occupation, as well as any other dietary, environmental or lifestyle factors you can think of that might have exposed that person to a disease-causing agent. Ask your family members about exposure history as well, for certain diseases such as mesothelioma, a rare form of lung cancer, is almost always associated with long term exposure to asbestos, often at work.

Another important factor to consider is how close the genetic relationship is between you and your affected relatives. As you probably already understand, the closer they are to you, the more likely it is that you may share the genetic factors that contributed to your relative's disease. Keep in mind, however, that even if a first-degree relative (parent, brother, sister) has a critical risk-increasing allele in one of his/her genes, there is no more than a 50% chance that you will inherit that particular genetic risk factor[2].

Table 4-1 illustrates the degree to which relatives share their genes. If one of your parents possesses a risk-increasing allele of a gene, for example, you have a 50% chance of inheriting that copy of the gene, and a 50% chance of inheriting the other copy of the gene that parent possesses. Siblings (brothers and sisters) share approximately half their genes, so if your brother or sister has inherited a risk-increasing gene allele from one of your parents, you have a 50% chance of having inherited that genetic factor as well. The risk gets lower as the distance between you and the affected relative increases.

Table 4-1. The chance of you possessing the risk-increasing gene alleles your affected family member has depends on how closely related you are.

This pair of relatives	Share this percentage of their genes
Identical twins	100 (except somatic mutations)
Fraternal (non-identical) twins	50
Parent-child	50
Siblings (brothers and sisters)	50
Grandparent-grandchild	25
Aunt/uncle-nephew/niece	25
First cousins	12.5
Great grandparent-great grandchild	12.5

---

[2]   This is true for the genes in your nucleus' DNA. As discussed above, however, mitochondrial mutations show a different pattern of inheritance. You will not inherit any mitochondrial mutations your father possesses, but will always inherit the mitochondrial mutations your mother possesses.

For most of the common multifactorial diseases, it often takes decades for an individual whose genes have provided him/her the typical level of protection to accumulate enough of a nongenetic load to overcome his/her defenses and make him/her sick. If an individual has a high genetic load, however, the individual's proteins do not provide him/her the usual level of protection against one or more disease-causing agents, so it doesn't take as much time for him/her to accumulate a nongenetic load that is heavy enough for the combined genetic and nongenetic loads to cause one of the corresponding diseases. When someone is diagnosed with a multifactorial disease at an unusually young age, this often means that the individual had a considerable genetic load for that disease. For example, because the average age for a woman to be diagnosed with breast cancer in the general population is age 65, if you have a female relative who was diagnosed with breast cancer when she was 85 (and there is no other family cancer history and no other personal risk factors), there is less concern about your genetic risk than there would be if she had been diagnosed with breast cancer at age 40.

The severity of the individual's disease can also sometimes give a clue as to the level of genetic factors that were involved in that particular case. Cancers, for example, can develop at one site in the body (a single primary cancer), or in multiple sites (more than one primary cancer, not cancer that has spread from the initial tumor). If the individual possesses a version of a protein that does not protect him/her well from a particular disease-causing agent, all the tissues in which that protein is not working so well will be susceptible to that disease-causing agent. In someone who has a heavy genetic load, the relevant tissues are susceptible enough that even a light nongenetic load will cause the person to have the disease. Because the heavy genetic load causes the tissues to be more susceptible from birth, it will be easier for the disease to appear in multiple places on the person's body. If a relative had both breast and ovarian cancer, and each was a new primary cancer (not spread from one site in the body to another, referred to as metastasis), you would have a greater genetic risk than you would if she had only had breast cancer, especially if the breast cancer developed at the same age as most cases do (60-70s).

Some of the multifactorial diseases appear more frequently in one sex than the other. For these diseases, the nongenetic factors appear to cause one sex to be more susceptible to the disease than the other sex is. If the disease is one that affects one sex more frequently or more severely than the next, the sex of your affected family members will influence your risk of developing the disease. For example, pyloric stenosis (PS) is an overgrowth of the muscles at the juncture between the stomach and small intestine. This can be life-threatening at birth and must be corrected by surgery or the newborn will not be able to digest foods. PS occurs five times more often in newborn boys than in newborn girls. The reason for this is unknown, but it is known that if you have an affected brother, your risk of having PS is 3.8%. If you have an affected sister, on the other hand, your risk of having PS is 9.2%.

A Quick Review Before We Go On

- Your family history is often an important source of information about your risk for specific diseases. When you compile your family history data, be sure to include as much as you can about the dietary, environmental and lifestyle factors that may have contributed to your affected family members' diseases. Obtaining medical records and death certificates on family members can help to clarify medical conditions and causes of death.

- The Surgeon General's office maintains a website (https://familyhistory.hhs.gov/fhh-web/home.action) called My Family Health Portrait, which enables you to generate a printable family pedigree.

- Having a close relative, even a parent, who is affected with a multifactorial disease does not guarantee that you will get the disease yourself. There are a number of reasons why you might not inherit the genetic factors that contributed to a disease in a close relative, even one of your parents. In addition, if nongenetic factors contributed strongly to your parent's disease, not only will you not inherit them, but you may be able to avoid them entirely.

- In most cases, the more affected relatives you have, the higher your genetic risk is, unless the affected relatives were all exposed to some critical nongenetic factor(s) that you are not exposed to.

- If you have a relative who is affected with a multifactorial disease, the more closely related you are, the higher your genetic risk may be.

- If your affected family members developed their diseases at earlier ages than most people do, this suggests that your genetic risk for that disease is high.

- Some multifactorial diseases affect one sex more frequently than the other. In these cases, the sex of your affected relatives will affect your level of risk.

Internet Websites That Can Help You Assess Your Risk For Cancer And Heart Disease

Your doctor or genetic counselor is the person who is best able to provide an accurate estimate of your genetic risk for one of the diseases that runs in your family. Some medical centers are developing websites that enable you to take an active role in this process yourself, however, and make it easier for you to gather and present the relevant information to your health care team. With the help of these websites, and your understanding of the principles we discuss in this book, you and your health care providers can better estimate what your genetic risk is for some of the diseases that have appeared in your family. At this time, the available websites focus on cancer and heart disease, for several reasons. These are the two most common medical causes of death in the U.S. In addition, if someone is found to have an increased genetic risk for one of these diseases, there are specific recommendations that can be made to reduce his/her exposure to several critical nongenetic factors, and thereby reduce his/her overall risk of developing the disease. Finally, there are several procedures available that may be able to detect the disease in its early stages, when it is easier to treat or cure.

Much Of The Current Focus Is On Nongenetic Factors

Some of the Internet websites that are currently available only consider nongenetic factors when they assess your risk for cancer and heart disease, while others use some limited family history data as well. As the field develops, however, these programs will incorporate more nongenetic factors, more complete family history data, clinical data such as blood sugar or cholesterol levels, and your status for critical gene variants as well. At this point in time, although a number of informative gene polymorphisms have been identified, little is known regarding the way these gene variants interact with other gene variants, or with dietary, environmental or lifestyle factors to influence your overall risk of developing the disease. In fact, one recent study of almost 12,000 women by the National Cancer Institute found that supplementing traditional risk factors (whether first-degree relatives such as a mother or sister developed breast cancer; reproductive history) with 10 genetic variants that have been shown to be associated with breast cancer did not improve the ability to estimate a woman's risk for breast cancer. As researchers learn more about the role our genes play in maintaining our health, however, they will become better able to use the results of genetic tests to improve the formulas by which they calculate disease risks.

Among the nongenetic factors, age is the most important factor that influences a woman's risk of developing breast cancer. At 35, most women have a 1 in 600 chance of developing breast cancer. By 50, however, the average woman's risk is 1 in 50 (2%). By 65, the risk has increased to 1 in 20 (5%). Hormones and reproductive factors play a significant role as well. Higher rates of breast cancer are associated with early menarche (first menstrual period), late menopause and either having a child after age 40 or never having given birth. Women who have more than three children also seem to have a reduced risk for breast cancer. The use of estrogen supplements, often as a hormone replacement for menopausal women, can increase the risk of breast cancer significantly, especially if taken for an extended period of time.

There are several nongenetic factors that have been shown to exert an important influence on your risk for heart disease as well. You cannot control some of these factors, such as your age and sex. You do have some level of control over several of the important factors, however. For example, you have a great deal of control over factors such as the level of fat in your diet, whether you smoke or not, your weight and the amount of exercise you get. You can also exert some amount of control over your blood pressure, the amount of stress you are exposed to and the level of fats in your blood. As the field of personalised medicine develops, programs that estimate your risk for heart disease will take more of these nongenetic factors into account.

The Family Health*Link* Program From The Ohio State University Medical Center

One of the medical centers that are leading the effort to help people understand their risks for common multifactorial diseases is the Ohio State University Medical Center. They maintain a website called Family Health*Link* (https://familyhealthlink.osumc. edu/), which can help you determine whether you have an average, moderate or high risk for cancer and/or heart disease. It is free to the public, and very easy to use. For each of your family members who has been diagnosed with cancer and/or heart disease, you simply put in your relationship to the affected family member, and the age at which he/she was diagnosed with the disease. Once you have entered information on all the relevant family members, the program automatically assesses the risk and provides you a printable report that you can share with your doctor. The report tells you whether your risk for cancer and heart disease is average, moderate or high, and discusses things you can do with respect to your diet, environment and lifestyle to reduce your overall risk of developing cancer or heart disease. People whose family history suggests that they have a high risk for cancer and/or heart disease are advised to see a genetic counselor or genetic specialist, to determine whether there are any genetic tests that may help their health care providers more accurately estimate their risk of developing cancer, as well as the risks faced by their family members.

As we discussed above, the age at which your affected members were diagnosed with their disease is an important factor that determines your genetic risk for these diseases. For example, imagine that Carmen, a 53-year-old woman whose mother, maternal aunt (mother's sister) and maternal grandmother (mother's mother) were all diagnosed with breast cancer, uses the Family Health*Link* program to estimate her genetic risk for breast cancer (Figure 4.4).

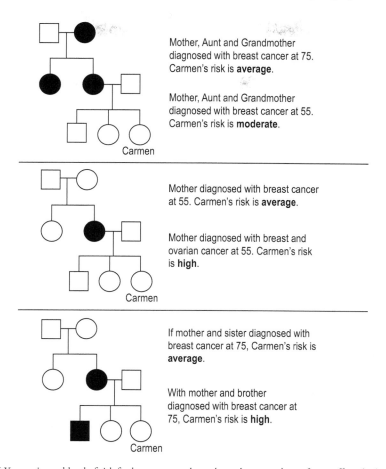

Mother, Aunt and Grandmother diagnosed with breast cancer at 75. Carmen's risk is **average**.

Mother, Aunt and Grandmother diagnosed with breast cancer at 55. Carmen's risk is **moderate**.

Mother diagnosed with breast cancer at 55. Carmen's risk is **average**.

Mother diagnosed with breast and ovarian cancer at 55. Carmen's risk is **high**.

If mother and sister diagnosed with breast cancer at 75, Carmen's risk is **average**.

With mother and brother diagnosed with breast cancer at 75, Carmen's risk is **high**.

Figure 4.4 Your estimated level of risk for breast cancer depends on the age and sex of your affected relatives.

Figure 4.4 illustrates how factors such as the age of diagnosis, the number of primary cancer sites and the sex of your affected relatives each affects your risk for breast cancer in its own way. If her mother, aunt and grandmother were all diagnosed with breast cancer at age 75, Carmen has an average risk for breast cancer based on her family history alone. It may surprise you that, with three close relatives affected with the same disease, her risk is only average. Because her relatives all developed cancer in their 70's, however, there is a good chance that nongenetic factors were more strongly involved than genetic factors in causing these women's cancers. If her mother, aunt and grandmother had all been diagnosed with breast cancer at age 55, Carmen's risk for breast cancer would increase to moderate (Figure 4.4, top panel).

One optimistic note is that, despite the fact that Carmen has three close relatives who were diagnosed with breast cancer at age 55, her risk is still only in the moderate range. As discussed above, there are a number of reasons why Carmen may not have inherited all of the genetic factors that her family members who have breast cancer may possess. People often overestimate their risk for a disease that has appeared in a family member, either because they overestimate the probability that they will inherit whatever genetic factors contributed to the relative's disease, or they underestimate the role that somatic mutations, mitochondrial mutations and avoidable nongenetic factors play in causing the disease.

As discussed above, having a relative with primary cancers in multiple sites increases your risk (Figure 4.4, middle panel). For example, if Carmen's mother was diagnosed with breast cancer at 55, and Carmen had no other affected relatives, Carmen's risk for breast cancer is average. However, if Carmen's mother was diagnosed with both breast and ovarian cancer at 55 years of age, and Carmen had no other affected relatives, Carmen's risk for breast and ovarian (possibly other cancers) becomes high. When someone develops primary cancers[3] in multiple places, this suggests that genetic factors played a strong role in causing the cancer, as they often do in the hereditary breast ovarian cancer syndrome (HBOC). We will discuss HBOC in more detail later in this chapter, and the genetic testing that is involved with this disease.

Finally, Figure 4.4 illustrates how important the gender of the affected relative can be in determining your risk for cancer, if it is a type of cancer that affects one sex more frequently than the other (Figure 4.4, bottom panel). As the figure illustrates, if Carmen's mother and sister were both diagnosed with breast cancer (which affects women more often than men) at age 55, Carmen's risk for breast cancer is moderate. If, however, her mother and brother were diagnosed with breast cancer at age 55, Carmen's risk for breast cancer is high. Even if her father and brother were diagnosed at age 75, Carmen's risk for breast cancer is still high. Contrast that with the fact that, if her mother and sister were diagnosed with breast cancer at age 75, Carmen's risk is only average. On the other hand, if Carmen's relatives were affected with colon cancer, which affects men and women with approximately equal frequency, her risk for colon cancer is the same whether it was her mother and sister who were affected with it, or her mother and brother.

The National Cancer Institute's Website

The National Cancer Institute also maintains a website (http://www.nci.nih.gov) that enables you to estimate your risk for breast cancer. This website uses what researchers call the Gail model to predict your risk for breast cancer. The Gail model provides an

---

[3]   "Primary cancer" refers to a cancer that originally arises at that site, as opposed to a metastasised cancer, which arose in another place and migrated to that site.

estimate of your risk of developing breast cancer within your lifetime, using several nongenetic factors, including age of first menstrual period, age at menopause, if you have had a prior breast biopsy and if the pathology was atypical, and whether there is a history of breast cancer in your parents, siblings or children.

The Gail model is useful for predicting your risk for breast cancer. Like all models, however, it has its limitations. The most important limitation of the Gail model stems from the fact that it only takes into account whether your close family members have developed breast cancer. If you have affected relatives other than your parents, siblings or children, the Gail model will not incorporate this information into its calculation, and therefore may underestimate your risk. It also does not take into account the age at which your affected relatives were diagnosed, or whether ovarian or other less common cancers run in a family. It also does not consider a person's ethnic heritage, which may affect his/her risk for hereditary forms of breast cancer.

Online Programs That Estimate Your Risk For Heart Disease

Twin and family studies have long shown that heart disease runs in families. In fact, family history contributes to your risk independently of other established risk-increasing factors such as high LDL cholesterol, low HDL cholesterol and diabetes. Approximately three out of every four people with early-onset heart disease (prior to age 55 years in men, prior to age 65 years in women) have a family history of heart disease. Having a close relative with early onset heart disease approximately doubles a person's risk. Having two or more first-degree relatives (parents, siblings or children) with heart disease increases a person's risk 3- to 6 times. In addition, having a brother or sister with heart disease appears to be a greater risk factor than having a parent with heart disease. The sex of your affected relatives also influences your risk. Having more than one female relative with heart disease in a family is more often associated with a greater genetic burden than having multiple affected male relatives is, and elevates the estimated risk for all family members. Identifying individuals and families who have a high risk for early onset heart disease is important, because there are a number of steps you can take to lower your risk of developing heart disease.

The Framingham Risk Score was developed from the Framingham Heart Study (http://www.framinghamheartstudy.org/risk/atrial.html#), and is often used to predict heart disease risk. The study began in 1948 with 5,209 adult participants from Framingham, Massachusetts, and is now on its third generation of participants. The purpose of the study was to follow a large group of unaffected people in a single community over time to identify common risk factors that contribute to heart disease.

Over the years, the Framingham Heart Study has led to the identification of many of the significant heart disease risk factors that we know of today, such as high blood pressure, high LDL cholesterol and triglycerides, age, gender, smoking, obesity, diabetes and physical inactivity. The online Framingham risk model takes into account many of these nongenetic risk factors in calculating a person's risk. However, it does not include family history, and therefore will likely underestimate heart disease risk for those with a significant family history.

A second online program, known as the CardioSmart Risk Assessment Tool (http://www.cardiosmart.org) also uses findings from the Framingham Heart Study. It is a very useful educational tool that predicts risk for developing a heart attack or dying from coronary disease (diseases of the blood vessels) within the next ten years. It is best used for people aged 20 years or older who do not have any form of heart disease or diabetes at that time. CardioSmart was designed by the American College of Cardiology.

Another program that enables you to estimate your risk for heart disease is the Reynolds Risk Score (http://www.reynoldsriskscore.org). The Reynolds Risk Score for women was developed by assessing 35 risk factors in 24,558 initially healthy American women who were followed for more than 10 years. This was part of the larger Women's Health Study, which was sponsored by the National Heart, Lung, and Blood Institute. The Reynolds Risk Score for men was developed using data from more than 10,000 initially healthy non-diabetic American men who were followed over a ten-year period for the development of heart attack, stroke, angioplasty, bypass surgery or death related to heart disease. The Reynolds Risk Score tool is more complete than CardioSmart, in that it also considers your level of a blood protein known as C-reactive protein, as well as whether your parents were diagnosed with heart disease prior to age 60.

Your Disease Risk (http://www.yourdiseaserisk.wustl.edu) also assesses your heart disease risk. This program considers your medical history, whether you smoke, some of your dietary habits, your level of physical activity and whether any of your first-degree relatives have had heart disease in its calculations.

Lastly, the Family Health*Link* program described above (https://familyhealthlink.osumc.edu) is also able to assess your risk for heart disease. It allows you to enter all family members with heart disease, on both sides of the family, as well as their age at diagnosis. The program then computes whether you have a high, moderate or low (compared to the general population) risk for heart disease. You can save and print the assessment to bring to your healthcare team. Those people at high or moderate risk are advised to meet with or speak to a genetic counselor to learn more about how the family history impacts risk and what they can do.

A Genetic Counselor Can Help You In Many Ways

Although your family doctor can provide basic risk assessment using personal and family medical history, more detailed analysis and assessment is at times necessary. In these cases, it may be helpful to meet with a genetic counselor for consultation. The National Society of Genetic Counselors offers a searchable directory of genetic counselors (http://www.nsgc.org/resourcelink.cfm). You can search by city, name, area of practice and zip code.

Genetic consultation is a health service that provides information and support to people who have, or may be at risk for, common and rare diseases. It is an important part of the decision-making process for genetic testing, and helps people better understand their risk for disease based on their personal and family medical history. In addition to attempting to determine your level of genetic risk, the genetic counselor will also ask about nongenetic influences such as dietary, environmental and lifestyle risk factors.

Genetic consultation is typically provided by a genetic counselor with an advanced degree, who at times also works with a geneticist (a doctor who specialises in genetics). Genetic counselors and geneticists have completed certified training and board examinations. Like other medical specialists' services, the consultation and risk assessment service is covered by most health insurance companies. Some insurance plans require a physician referral.

Genetic consultations may take place in a hospital, genetic center or other type of medical center or office. Phone consultations and even virtual consultations are becoming more available as well. The genetic professional will review your personal medical history, your family history (using a four-generation pedigree), and ask questions about your diet, environment and lifestyle. The consultation may also include a targeted physical examination. The genetic professional will also explain the basic genetic and medical issues involved and address any questions you may have. If you have a family history of a single-gene disease, the genetic professional will explain the expected pattern of inheritance for that disease, estimate the potential risk for you and other family members, and will present you with the options for testing and treatment. If you have a family history of a multifactorial disease, the genetic professional will provide you with the most accurate estimate possible of your risk. He/she may also recommend genetic testing, changes to your diet, environment or lifestyle, or that you have some type of screening test performed.

If you are considering having genetic/genomic testing performed, or are wondering if this testing will benefit you, a genetic counselor can discuss the benefits, limitations and risks associated with the testing, and help you make an informed decision. Despite the fact that genetic/genomic tests will grow increasingly more useful in the near future, they will always have limitations, and it will always be necessary to consider the limitations as well as the potential benefits of any given genetic test. Genetic counseling also allows you the opportunity to anticipate the emotional or psychological consequences the test results might have for you or your family members. You should discuss what your reaction will be to a positive, negative or inconclusive result, and the possible effects these results may have on other family members. Prior to any test, you should also have a clear understanding of what screening or prevention measures you may be able to take if the test indicates that you have a relatively high genetic risk, as well as what treatment options are available if you already have the disease.

In addition to these issues, the confidentiality and privacy of results must be addressed, and issues of employment and insurance discrimination require careful discussion. The genetic counselor will try to detect and respond to any unspoken fears or questions you may have, but being as open as you can be about your concerns will insure that you get as much benefit out of the counseling experience as possible.

The genetic counselor will obtain your informed consent, and arrange to get preauthorisation from your insurance company, if your insurance provider is going to cover the cost of testing. Any blood or other samples that are necessary for testing will then be taken. Once the results of the test are available, the genetic counselor will discuss the results of the testing and help you cope with any anxiety or psychological distress you may feel. The counselor may recommend that you undergo screening tests regularly, or recommend changing certain aspects of your diet, environment or lifestyle to help lower your risk of developing the disease. The counselor may also recommend that certain family members be tested as well. In addition, the option to participate in research studies is offered when appropriate.

You will receive quite a lot of information during a genetic counseling session; between the amount of information and the fact that you may be experiencing strong emotions at the time, do not be surprised if it is hard to process it all. For this reason, a detailed summary letter is usually provided to the patient and their healthcare providers, to outline and review the important issues and describe the plan for the future. The genetic counselor can also refer you to the appropriate professionals if you need more intensive psychosocial or family counseling.

Once you establish a relationship with a genetic counselor, you should remain in touch with him/her periodically. Given the fast pace at which the field is advancing, you may want to ask the counselor once in a while if there have been any recent advances in personalised medicine testing that could benefit you. This also allows you to update your family history data periodically; family and medical histories change over time, and these changes may affect the risk assessment and/or management plan.

JENNIFER'S STORY: *BRCA1* AND *BRCA2* GENETIC TESTING FOR HEREDITARY BREAST-OVARIAN CANCER SYNDROME (HBOC)

Jennifer is 28, in generally good health, but she is worried about her risk for breast and ovarian cancer. Although there was no formal medical record to document it, Jennifer had always been told that her maternal grandmother (her mother's mother) had died from a "female" cancer in her early 50s. Jennifer's maternal aunt Mary (her mother's sister) had been diagnosed with breast cancer when she was 38. Mary is now 53. She has had multiple tumors in one of her breasts, and had chosen to have a double mastectomy (surgical removal of both breasts). Because her mother was thought to have died of a "female" cancer, Mary also had surgery to remove her ovaries, because she had been told this would decrease her chances of developing ovarian cancer. Jennifer's mother Sarah is currently 50, and is unaffected, but has not had a mammogram or clinical breast examination in four years. Jennifer's pedigree is illustrated in Figure 4.5

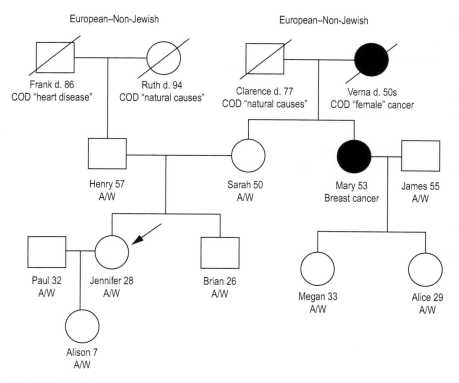

Figure 4.5 Jennifer's pedigree. People's current ages or ages at death are indicated next to their names. A/W = alive and well; COD = cause of death

Making The Decision Whether Or Not To Have Testing

The fact that Jennifer's Aunt Mary developed breast cancer at such an early age and had multiple tumors, along with the strong possibility of ovarian cancer in Jennifer's grandmother, suggests there is a reasonable probability that a risk-increasing gene allele for these cancers may be present in the family. Jennifer's family history suggests that the family may have hereditary breast ovarian cancer syndrome (HBOC). This syndrome is caused by germline mutations in either the *BRCA1* or *BRCA2* gene. Genetic testing is available for both genes. Jennifer is having a hard time deciding whether or not to have genetic testing, though.

Jennifer is experiencing a number of emotions, some of them conflicting. Because her maternal aunt and grandmother both had advanced cancer at a relatively young age, Jennifer is very anxious about the prospect of getting tested, because she expects the test to tell her she possesses a risk-increasing gene allele. While Jennifer also feels that knowing she faces a fate like Mary's would be a great psychological burden, she also knows that if there is a critical risk-increasing allele running in her family, genetic testing is the only way for her to know whether she has it, and whether she might have passed it down to her 7-year old daughter, Alison.

Jennifer also understands that being told you have a risk-increasing gene allele for HBOC does not automatically constitute a death sentence. Jennifer has talked to her gynecologist, as well as read several articles that illustrate how regular clinical breast examinations and screening tests such as mammograms can detect cancers as they begin to develop, and increase the chances for successful treatment if breast cancer is found at an early stage. Because she is aware of the benefits of such screening procedures, Jennifer is more comfortable than her mother is with the prospect of getting regular breast examinations and beginning these at an earlier age than is recommended for women who have a typical level of risk.

Jennifer's greatest concern is not about her prospects for breast cancer; she is more concerned about her chances for developing ovarian cancer. She has learned that modern-day screening procedures are not nearly as effective at detecting ovarian cancer as they are at detecting breast cancer. Because of the limitations of modern-day ovarian cancer screening procedures, Jennifer is very frightened by the thought that the only way she may be able to prevent the development of ovarian cancer is to have a preventive surgery and have her ovaries and fallopian tubes removed.

Jennifer's First Visit With The Genetic Counselor

Jennifer decides that the benefits of getting tested outweigh the potential negative effects, and decides to seek genetic testing. She has read newspaper articles about the *BRCA* genes, and she knows that some alleles of *BRCA1* and *BRCA2* increase a woman's risk for developing breast and ovarian cancer. Jennifer also goes on the Internet, and finds several companies that offer whole-genome SNP screens directly to consumers. She spends some time digesting the information about what whole-genome SNP screens do and what benefits they can provide. The information she reads on the testing companies' websites makes it clear that these tests provide the consumer a great deal of information, some of which has implications for your health and health care. Jennifer is confused, however, by the fact that these websites all also include a disclaimer that says the information that these tests provide is not intended to aid in medical diagnoses or help a doctor make decisions about medical treatments. Jennifer decides to make an appointment with a genetic counselor, to ask the many questions she has about genetic testing, and to discuss the potential benefits and limitations of the tests that are available.

The meeting with the genetic counselor takes approximately two hours. They go through Jennifer's medical and family history in detail and discuss the testing options. The counselor is familiar with the whole-genome SNP screens that Jennifer has read about, and informs Jennifer that the whole-genome SNP screen will provide her with a lot of information, but very little of that information is relevant to Jennifer's risk for cancer. Very few of the SNPs that are included in the whole-genome SNP screens that are currently available influence a woman's risk for breast and/or ovarian cancer. In addition, two of the most important genes to test in Jennifer's case, the *BRCA1* and *BRCA2* genes that have been associated with HBOC, are not included in the whole-genome SNP panels, because the company that developed the tests for *BRCA1* and *BRCA2* variants has patented the sequence of the *BRCA1* and *BRCA2* genes[4].

The genetic counselor informs Jennifer that the most useful test for her at this time will be the tests that detect sequence variations in the *BRCA1* and *BRCA2* genes. Because researchers have found thousands of risk-increasing alleles in the *BRCA1* and *BRCA2* genes by now, a complete sequencing of the two genes is the only way to determine which risk-increasing alleles any given person has. The test is done on either a blood or saliva sample. Although many of the larger insurance plans provide coverage for the test, they usually require the person to meet certain eligibility criteria, such as having been diagnosed with breast cancer before age 45. Because Jennifer does not meet her insurance carrier's criteria, her insurance company will not pay for these tests, which can cost $3400 or more. Jennifer feels, however, that the information the test will provide is worth the cost, and decides to proceed with testing.

To help prepare Jennifer to receive the results of her test, the counselor also reviews the possible test results that Jennifer might receive. The counselor knows that it is especially important to prepare Jennifer for the possibility she may be told that she has

---

[4] Note that a federal court ruled on March 29, 2010 that the Myriad company's patents on the *BRCA1* and *BRCA2* genes are invalid. However, the case will probably be appealed, and there are other events that must occur to enable other companies to include the *BRCA1* and *BRCA2* genes in their tests. This ruling is unlikely to have any immediate impact on the availability of *BRCA* gene testing.

a risk-increasing allele of either the *BRCA1* or *BRCA2* gene, and help her understand exactly how possessing one of these risk-increasing alleles will influence her risk of developing cancer.

The counselor explains that the general population risk for developing breast cancer by age 40 is 1%, and the lifetime breast cancer risk for women in general is 10-12%. In contrast, however, the risk of developing breast cancer for a woman with either a *BRCA1* or *BRCA2* mutation is 60-80% over her lifetime. In addition, a woman who possesses a *BRCA1* or *BRCA2* gene mutation has an increased risk of developing breast cancer by her mid-20's, and should begin undergoing intensive breast cancer screening by at least age 25. By age 40, approximately 15% of women who carry *BRCA1* mutations will have already developed their first breast cancer. This rises to 28% by age 50. In women with *BRCA2* mutations, the risks are at least 5% by age 40 and 13% by age 50.

The counselor also explains that a woman who has already had breast cancer and who has a *BRCA* mutation also has a 40-60% risk of developing a second breast cancer over the remainder of her lifetime. The risk of developing ovarian or fallopian tube cancer is also increased considerably. This is a rather rare cancer in the general population (1% risk over the lifetime for most people). However, for *BRCA1* or *BRCA2* mutation carriers, the risk for ovarian cancer is 15-60% over their lifetime. The age of onset of ovarian cancer for *BRCA* variant carriers is also much earlier (mid to late 30s) than the age of onset in the general population (mid-60s).

The counselor also reminds Jennifer of the importance of nongenetic factors in causing cancers. The counselor explains that the course of the disease is highly variable in women who have risk-increasing alleles of *BRCA1* or *BRCA2*. Some develop multiple cancers before age 50, while others are still cancer-free at 70. The fact that the course of the disease is so variable illustrates the importance of other genetic or nongenetic factors in the development of the disease. The counselor discusses several of the nongenetic factors that may influence a woman's risk for breast or ovarian cancer. For example, the use of birth control pills has been shown to significantly lower ovarian cancer risk in *BRCA* mutation carriers. Not smoking may also help reduce risk. This information also helps reduce some of Jennifer's anxiety.

The counselor also informs Jennifer that, even if the test reveals no risk-increasing alleles in *BRCA1* or *BRCA2*, this does not necessarily mean that Jennifer has an overall low risk for developing breast cancer. The counselor points out that *BRCA1* and *BRCA2* are only two of many genes that influence a woman's risk for breast cancer. In fact, only 5-7% of women with breast cancer have a risk-increasing allele in either *BRCA1* or *BRCA2*, and only 10-15% of women with ovarian cancer have a risk-increasing allele in either *BRCA1* or *BRCA2*. If Jennifer's Aunt Mary's cancer did not involve a critical risk-increasing *BRCA1* or *BRCA2* gene allele, it remains possible that another, still undiscovered, breast cancer gene(s) may have been involved. In addition, many of the nongenetic factors that contribute to breast cancer are still unknown.

Finally, the genetic counselor informs Jennifer that the wisest testing strategy would begin with testing Jennifer's Aunt Mary, rather than Jennifer herself. The counselor tells Jennifer that approximately 10-15% of people who have complete *BRCA1/BRCA2* testing receive a report stating that a variant was found in the gene's sequence, but the analysts cannot be certain whether this variant is expected to alter the level of activity in the protein. Because of the possible uncertainty in the interpretation of the results, it is best to begin by testing someone who has or has had breast or ovarian cancer. Ideally, it is best to test the family member who was diagnosed at the earliest age, if possible. If Aunt Mary is found to have a risk-increasing allele in one of the *BRCA* genes, then Jennifer can have a test performed that specifically determines whether she also possesses that same allele. This would be the most informative test. Moreover, Aunt Mary has two daughters (who are also at risk because of their family history), and this information would be helpful to them. Jennifer decides to talk with her aunt and see if she would be interested in having the *BRCA* gene test.

Interpreting The Test Results

Jennifer's Aunt Mary sees a local genetic counselor and decides to have *BRCA* testing, which finds that a single nucleotide has been deleted from her *BRCA1* gene sequence. This sequence variant has been reported in other people already, and is known to be a risk-increasing allele for HBOC. The counselor informs Jennifer that the probability of Jennifer possessing the same risk-increasing allele is 25%, or 1 in 4. Jennifer then chooses to have testing for that *BRCA1* mutation, and when the test results come back, Jennifer learns that she does, indeed, have the same *BRCA1* allele that Mary has. Further, Jennifer is told that women who have this mutation have a 70% chance of developing breast cancer and a 40-60% risk of developing ovarian cancer in her lifetime.

In addition to their impact on Jennifer, Jennifer's test results also have implications for her mother Sarah and other family members. Jennifer could not have inherited the risk-increasing *BRCA1* allele directly from her Aunt Mary; she must have inherited it from her mother Sarah. Sarah is an **obligate carrier** of the risk-increasing allele; because her sister and daughter both have the allele, she must have it herself[5].

---

[5]   It is also technically possible that Sarah might not have the risk-increasing *BRCA1* allele, and that Jennifer might have inherited the risk-increasing *BRCA1* allele from her father. The fact that Jennifer's aunt has the risk-increasing *BRCA1* allele, however, and the fact that her father has no family history of any *BRCA*-related cancers makes this highly unlikely.

Jennifer's test results also have important implications for her 26-year-old brother Brian. Although women are more likely to actually develop breast cancer, within any given family, risk-increasing alleles of *BRCA1* and *BRCA2* are seen as frequently in men as they are in women. As Jennifer appears to have inherited the risk-increasing allele from her mother, then her brother Brian has a 50% chance of having inherited that same allele as well. Men with a *BRCA* mutation face increased cancer risks, specifically for male breast cancer and prostate cancer. A typical male's risk for breast cancer is less than 1% over the course of a lifetime. In contrast, the risk for male breast cancer for men who carry *BRCA2* mutations is approximately 5-6% over the course of a lifetime, with less risk for *BRCA1* carriers. The degree of prostate cancer risk varies between *BRCA1* and *BRCA2* carriers, with most studies suggesting a two- to three-fold increase over the general population risk of 10-12%, or approximately 20-36% risk for prostate cancer over a lifetime. There is also some increased risk in men and women with *BRCA2* mutations for skin melanoma and pancreatic cancer, and possibly other cancers as well.

Designing Personalised Healthcare Plans For Jennifer, Her Mother And Her Daughter

Although Jennifer is somewhat dismayed at finding that she possesses the risk-increasing *BRCA1* allele, her most immediate concern is for her mother, Sarah. She explains to her mother that her test result makes it highly likely that Sarah has the risk-increasing *BRCA1* allele as well. While she cannot convince her mother to have the genetic testing performed, she does convince her to make an appointment for a mammogram and a clinical breast examination. Sarah is found to have an early stage breast cancer.

Upon realising that she has developed cancer, Sarah gets very anxious about her future, and somewhat depressed as well. Because her daughter and sister have the risk-increasing *BRCA1* allele, she understands that she must also have it, too. She also understands that having this *BRCA1* gene allele increases her risk of developing additional primary cancers as well. She discusses these matters with her doctor, and also speaks with the genetic counselor. Sarah chooses not only to have the breast with the detectable tumors removed, but the other one as well, to prevent cancer from developing in that breast. This procedure decreases the risk of developing a new breast cancer by 90-95% in women who carry risk-increasing alleles in *BRCA1* or *BRCA2*

Because Sarah also has a high risk for ovarian cancer, Sarah is referred by her doctor to meet with a specialist to discuss preventive surgery approaches once she completes her breast cancer treatments. Sarah is also referred to a psychiatrist to help with the psychological issues that she is experiencing.

With respect to Jennifer's health care plan, the genetic counselor knows that the National Cancer Institute has recommended that women who have a high genetic risk for breast cancer should begin getting annual breast imaging, including mammograms and magnetic resonance imaging (MRI) studies, by age 25, or at 10 years younger than the earliest age at which an affected relative was diagnosed with breast cancer. In addition, they should have a clinical breast examination by a physician every six months, and perform monthly breast self-examinations. The counselor provides a referral to a comprehensive breast health clinic, which is staffed by breast specialists who can provide more comprehensive screening and preventive health care.

The genetic counselor also informs Jennifer that there are several support groups and Internet websites for women with risk-increasing alleles in the *BRCA* genes. For example, groups such as Facing Our Risk For Cancer Empowered (FORCE, http://www.facingourrisk.org/) and BE BRIGHT PINK (http://www.bebrightpink.org/) provide educational materials and psychological support for women who have high risk for breast and/or ovarian cancer.

Jennifer might also want to consider taking a preventive medication to reduce the risk of developing breast cancer. Both tamoxifen (sold as Nolvadex, Istubal, and Valodex) and raloxifene (Evista) may be effective in preventing breast cancer in women who possess risk-increasing alleles in either the *BRCA1* or *BRCA2* genes. The potential benefits of these drugs must be weighed against their side effects, however. The staff of the comprehensive breast health program will be able to advise Jennifer of the risks and benefits of the drugs.

In addition, the counselor notes that Jennifer's risk-increasing *BRCA1* allele also increases her risk for ovarian cancer. Jennifer has been on birth-control pills for seven years now, which has been shown in a few studies to reduce the risk of ovarian cancer by half for women who carry risk-increasing *BRCA* alleles. Further, Jennifer decides to undergo several procedures that can screen for ovarian cancer, including a pelvic examination, testing of a blood protein called CA-125, and a transvaginal ultrasound examination.

Because the current screening procedures for ovarian cancer have significant limitations, Jennifer is advised to consider the possibility of having her ovaries and Fallopian tubes removed around age 35, or after she has finished having children. This surgery will lower her risk for developing ovarian cancer by approximately 80-90%, and may also lower her risk for developing breast cancer by approximately 50%, dependent upon the age at which she has this preventive surgery. Jennifer is referred to a gynecologist who specialises in high-risk cases for consultation.

The counselor also informs Jennifer that, because one of her two copies of the *BRCA1* gene has the risk-increasing allele, her daughter Alison has a 50% chance of possessing the risk-increasing allele. Because Alison is 7, and because the increased cancer risk in *BRCA* carriers begins in early adulthood, Jennifer chooses to wait until she is older before discussing the issue with her. Because Alison will not reach reproductive age for several years, Jennifer can plan carefully, and even has time to expose Alison to educational materials that will allow Alison to feel even more comfortable than Jennifer did with the prospect of having genetic testing performed.

CHAPTER SUMMARY

- Your family medical history contains important information that can help you estimate your risk for the diseases that have affected your family members. The Surgeon General's My Family Health Portrait website can help you compile your family's medical history, as well as information about nongenetic factors that might have contributed to your affected family members' diseases, so you can present the information to your health care providers.

- Even if you have a close relative who has a disease, you may not have a high risk of developing that disease. You may not have the other critical gene variants, or may not have been exposed to the critical nongenetic factors.

- The number of affected relatives you have, their specific relation to you, the ages at which they developed their diseases, and sometimes their sex, all influence your risk for those diseases.

- Several Internet websites contain programs that can help you estimate your risk for cancer and heart disease.

- There are many ways in which a genetic counselor can help you. A counselor can help you collect and interpret your family history information, and determine if there are any changes you can make to your diet, environment or lifestyle that will reduce your risk of developing specific diseases. A genetic counselor can also help you understand the potential benefits and limitations of genetic testing, and cope with the psychological and emotional stress that you may feel because of the diseases that run in your family or the possibility that a genetic/genomic test may reveal that you have a high genetic risk for a specific disease.

CHAPTER 5

USING GENETIC TESTING TO MAINTAIN YOUR HEALTH AND PERSONALISE YOUR MEDICAL CARE, NOW AND IN THE FUTURE

THE CURRENTLY AVAILABLE GENETIC TESTS PROVIDE A VARIETY OF SPECIFIC BENEFITS

Genetic tests are capable of providing a wide assortment of benefits, but it is important to remember that all genetic tests have significant limitations. In Chapter 6 we discuss some of the issues that are involved in interpreting the results of genetic tests, and describe the limitations of the genetic tests that are currently available. In this chapter, we build upon the principles discussed in Chapters 1-4, to help you understand what tests are available now, and how these tests provide you information about the level of activity of important proteins.

Some Tests Help Estimate Your Risk For Diseases

One way in which genetic testing will be used to help improve health care is to provide tests that accurately estimate your risk for specific diseases. Researchers can identify one or more places in the gene's sequence where the specific version of the sequence that the person possesses affects the protein's level of activity. A test can then be designed to determine whether the version(s) of the gene that a given person has increase or decrease his/her risk for the corresponding disease. These predictive tests can take one of two forms:

- There are a number of single-gene diseases (see Table III-1 for examples) for which predictive genetic tests are available.
- Some genetic tests help estimate your risk for specific multifactorial diseases.

Most of the single-gene diseases are rare, so testing for these diseases is usually done only when there is a strong indication that a disease-causing mutation might be found. Examples of situations in which these tests are appropriate include when there is a family history of the disease, if a child is born with the condition (i.e. cystic fibrosis), or if the person has a parent who has the disease.

Some single-gene diseases can be caused by a mutation in one of several genes, so it may require an analysis of several genes before the critical mutation is found. Once the causative mutation is found, this can provide more definitive information about the cause of disease (if the person is affected) or the probability the person will develop the disease later in life.

Because there are so many genes that influence your risk of developing any given multifactorial disease, each risk-increasing or risk-decreasing allele usually only has a small effect on your overall risk of developing the disease. In order to assess all the genetic factors that must be included to produce a reliable estimate of the person's risk of developing a multifactorial disease, it is usually necessary to analyse many more genes than must be analysed for the typical single-gene disease. At the present time, researchers have only discovered a small percentage of the genetic factors that influence your risk for any multifactorial disease. In addition, as we discussed in Chapter 1, one of the big challenges facing researchers is to determine exactly how to combine information about the risk-increasing and risk-decreasing alleles the person possesses with the other critical factors. The person's genetic information needs to be combined with information about nongenetic factors to produce a test that can accurately predict a person's risk of developing the disease. Some factors influence your risk more strongly than others. In addition, the critical genetic or nongenetic risk factors may not simply add together. They may multiply each other when they occur together, or interact even more dramatically than that.

Some Tests Screen Prospective Parents For Recessive Mutations

Some tests screen prospective parents to see if they carry gene mutations that can cause recessive genetic diseases. As we discussed in Chapter 3, it is well known that some single-gene diseases can be caused by the person having two copies of an autosomal recessive mutation, or a woman having two copies of an X-linked recessive mutation. The degree to which these recessive mutations contribute to multifactorial diseases is less well known, however. If you carry a recessive mutation, you have a 1 in 2 chance of passing it down to each of your children. If both parents carry a recessive mutation in the same gene, there is a 1 in 4 chance that the child will inherit both mutations, and have the associated recessive disease.

In addition, as we discussed in Chapter 1, the frequency of people who carry certain recessive mutations can be surprisingly high (see Table 5-1). Many people who have a family history of a recessive genetic disease want to know if they carry the mutation that runs in their family. Those who do carry their family's mutation often want their partners to be tested as well, to determine the probability that their child will develop the disease.

Table 5-1 Carrier Frequencies For Some Recessive Mutations

Disease	Gene Symbol and Name	Carrier Frequency and Population*
Cystic Fibrosis	*CFTR*; Cystic fibrosis transmembrane regulator	1/25 C; 1/150 As; 1/70 Af
Hemochromatosis	*HFE*; Hereditary hemochromatosis protein	1/10 C; 1/43 Af; 1/36 H
Alpha-1antitrypsin deficiency	*SERPINA1*; Serine protease inhibitor type A1	1/50 U
Spinal muscular atrophy	*SMN1*; Survival of motor neuron 1	1/50 U

* C = Caucasians, As = Asian-Americans, Af = African-Americans, H = Hispanic-Americans, U = Unspecified American population

Prenatal Testing Can Reveal Whether A Child Has Inherited A Parent's Mutation

Many people who carry mutations that are capable of causing disease are anxious about the possibility of passing the mutation down to one or more of their children. A sample of the fetus' DNA can be obtained by amniocentesis, in which some of the amniotic fluid in which the fetus is floating is removed. Amniotic fluid contains many skin cells that have fallen off the fetus. The fetus' DNA can be obtained from these skin cells, and analysed to see if the fetus has inherited the parent's mutation.

Some Tests Help Your Doctor Diagnose Your Condition And Personalise Your Medical Treatments

There are several ways in which genetic tests can help your doctor make an accurate diagnosis and choose the safest and most effective treatments for you. They include:

- Situations in which the symptoms of several diseases overlap each other, and it can be difficult for your doctor to determine exactly which of several possible diseases you have. In some cases, genetic testing can help the doctor diagnose a disease in someone who is showing symptoms that might indicate one of several diseases.

• Diseases for which there are several different drugs that can be prescribed. Some people will respond better to one drug than another, and researchers are working to develop genetic tests that can predict which drug will be best for you.

• Choosing the proper starting dose for you even when there is only one drug available to treat your disorder. There is a great deal of variability in the rate at which different people metabolise, or break down, a lot of prescription drugs. Genetic tests that determine how quickly your body will break down a prescription drug can help your doctor choose the best dose to prescribe for you.

In some cases, a genetic test that improves your doctor's ability to diagnose your disease may help your doctor quickly determine the safest and most effective treatment for you. In addition, tests that help doctors choose the safest and most effective drug doses for their patients will reduce the amount of time and money that get wasted because of ineffective treatments, and the number of people who get admitted to hospitals because of adverse drug reactions. Because pharmacology (the science of drug development and drug treatments) is such an important cornerstone of medicine, the fields of **pharmacogenetics** and **pharmacogenomics** are very active areas of research.

One of the fields of medicine in which pharmacogenetic and pharmacogenomic testing are improving the safety and effectiveness of medical treatments involves personalising drug therapy for people who have cancer. As a cancer progresses, the activity levels of a number of genes change in the cancerous cells. Not all people who have a given cancer experience the same changes in gene activity, however, which is one reason why there is so much variability in different people's responses to cancer therapies. A test that indicated whether an anti-cancer drug would be effective for a particular patient would allow a doctor to avoid prescribing a medication that would cause the patient to endure unpleasant or dangerous side effects without reaping any benefit from the drug.

For example, in approximately one-fourth of all invasive breast cancer cases, there is an increased level of activity in a gene called *HER2* in the tumor cells. The drug Herceptin can help these patients, but it will not help patients in whom the *HER2* gene is not overactive. Tests have been developed to determine whether the *HER2* gene is overactive in the tumor cells of a specific patient. Those patients whose *HER2* gene is not overactive can be spared the discomfort and danger associated with Herceptin's side effects.

Knowing whether certain genes' activities have changed may also allow the doctor to better predict whether someone is likely to develop cancer in a second site in his/her body. The Oncotype DX® test (Genomic Health, Inc.) and the MammaPrint test

(Agendia) determine the activity levels of a number of genes in the patient's cancerous cells, and can help predict the patient's risk for having cancer develop in another site in the body in the future. Patients with a low risk of recurrence may be best treated with drugs such as tamoxifen, and spared the dangerous and unpleasant side effects of the other chemotherapy drugs that are used to treat cancer patients.

Some of the changes that occur in cancerous cells involve structural rearrangements of the chromosomes themselves, *e.g.* deletions, different chromosomes exchanging pieces. For example, in 95% of patients who have chronic myelogenous leukemia, chromosomes 9 and 22 have exchanged pieces in the cancerous cells (this rearrangement is often referred to as the Philadelphia chromosome). Knowing whether the patient's cancerous cells possess this chromosome rearrangement can help the doctor decide whether to prescribe drugs such as Desatinib for that patient.

These and other research efforts in the fields of pharmacogenetics and pharmacogenomics show a lot of promise, but the initial efforts have been too restricted to achieve the best possible results. Most of the pharmacogenetic tests that are available today focus on genes whose proteins metabolise specific drugs, because that is the aspect of the process about which we know the most.

In order to get a complete assessment of the way our bodies will respond to a drug, however, you also have to consider how sensitive the target tissues and organs are to the drug. The drug's target tissue will be more sensitive to a given concentration of the drug in one person than in another. These aspects of the way our bodies handle drugs are harder to measure than the rate of drug metabolism. Determining the influence these gene variants have over your response to the drug may involve measuring the response of a particular tissue or protein to the drug in the laboratory, or measuring the rate at which the system the drug targets works in your body before and after you begin taking the drug.

It will take a little time before we identify the genes that influence all the different aspects of our responses to drugs. We already have the capability to answer many of the critical questions, however, and it will only be a short time before researchers develop tests that incorporate genes whose proteins metabolise the drug, genes whose proteins act as receptors for the drug in the body, and genes whose proteins regulate the normal activity of the molecules, tissues and systems that the drug targets.

Some Tests Provide Information That Is Of Personal, Rather Than Medical, Interest

Some of the genetic tests that are advertised directly to consumers provide information about items of purely personal interest. Some have even referred to this as a "recreational" use of genetic information. For example:

- Many of our physical and behavioral traits are multifactorial, and some of the tests that are advertised to consumers include gene variants that influence your chances of having certain normal traits. These tests can tell you such things as your chances of having red hair, or going bald, whether you can taste certain substances in food and drinks, and certain aspects of your personality.
- Some of these genetic tests provide information about your ancestry.

In most cases, the tests that look at genes that influence your normal traits merely provide explanations for things you already know about yourself. For example, a red-haired person may get a test report that says he/she has two gene alleles that increase your chances of having red hair.

These tests are subject to the same limitations as described above, however. They are far from complete, because a lot of the genetic factors that influence your normal traits have not been identified yet. The tests often look at one or a few relevant gene sites, but together these sites often only account for a small percentage of the genetic factors that influence these traits. Because of this, many people will find that they have one or more gene alleles that increase their risk for a specific trait, but they do not have that trait. This is presumably because they do not possess other critical genetic or nongenetic factors that increase your chances of having the trait.

Some people seek genetic testing to learn more about their ancestry. In most cases, what they find is consistent with things they already knew, but some people may learn interesting new facts about their genetic origins through these tests. The mitochondrial DNA that we discussed in Chapter 3 is commonly used for studies of ancestry. As we described, we inherit all of our mitochondrial DNA from our mother. Mitochondrial DNA therefore allows the testing laboratory to determine your mother's ancestral origins. Y chromosome sequences, on the other hand, are passed down from father to son, and can be used to trace your father's ancestry. Because women lack a Y chromosome, however, a woman would have to obtain material from her father to learn about that aspect of her ancestry.

THE TYPES OF DNA SEQUENCE VARIATIONS THAT ARE DETECTED BY GENETIC TESTS

In order to perform a genetic test, the testing laboratory must obtain a sample of one of the tissues or fluids from your body. If you obtain genetic testing through your doctor, your doctor will usually take a blood sample (your white blood cells contain DNA). In contrast, genetic testing companies that advertise directly to consumers will send you a tube into which you can deposit a saliva sample (saliva contains skin cells from the lining of your mouth). The laboratory then extracts the DNA from your cells, using a procedure that breaks up the cells' membranes, causing the cells to dump out their contents, including their DNA.

The sequence variations that most genetic tests look at take one of several forms. The effects that these sequence variants will have on the level of activity of their gene's protein can be predicted by applying the principles we discussed in Chapter 2. The four primary types of sequence variation these tests detect are:

- **Substitutions:** There are many places in our DNA sequence in which most people have one particular base in that position of the sequence (for example, an A), but some people have a different base there (either a C, G or T).
- **Duplications:** Sometimes an extra copy is made of a stretch of sequence, and the copied sequence is lying next to the original sequence.
- **Insertions:** Sometimes one or more bases that are usually found at a distant site in the DNA have been added to the sequence of a gene.
- **Deletions:** Sometimes one or more bases have been lost from the sequence of a gene.
- **Repeated Sequence Polymorphisms:** There are places in your DNA in which a stretch of sequence is repeated multiple times. The stretch of sequence that gets repeated can range from a single base to very long stretches of sequence (up to 1,000,000 bases). Different people will have a different number of repetitions of the repeated sequence, and the number of repetitions of the repeated sequence you have can sometimes influence the activity of a gene or its protein.

Base Substitutions May Or May Not Change The Protein's Amino Acid Sequence

Recall from Chapter 2 that there are at least 15 million SNPs in the human DNA sequence. As you can see in Figure 5.1, these single base substitutions may or may not change the amino acid sequence of the protein, depending on exactly how they change the sequence of the mRNA codon in which they lie. One reason why a single base substitution may not change the level of activity in the gene's protein is the fact that the genetic code (Figure 2.2) is redundant. There are many situations in which you can substitute one base for another in the mRNA and still have the protein contain the same sequence of amino acids.

"Normal" mRNA codon sequence	AUG Methionine	AUU Isoleucine	CCA Proline	GCC Alanine
Single nucleotide substitution, no amino acid change	AUG Methionine	AU**C** Isoleucine	CCA Proline	GCC Alanine
Single nucleotide substitution, causes amino acid change	AUG Methionine	AU**G** Methionine	CCA Proline	GCC Alanine
1 base deletion (U*), changes all codons after	A*GA Arginine	UGC Cysteine	CAG Glutamine	CC Proline
1 base insertion (U), changes all codons after	AU**U** Isoleucine	GAU Aspartic acid	UCC Serine	AGC Serine

3 base insertion (UUU), adds one amino acid	AUG Methionine	**UUU** Phenylalanine	AUU Isoleucine	CCA Proline	GCC Alanine

Figure 5.1. You can predict the effect a sequence variation will have on the gene's protein can be predicted by applying the principles that were discussed in Chapter 2.

In other situations, substituting one base for another can cause one amino acid to be substituted for another. As we discussed in Chapter 2, the effect this will have on the protein's activity depends on how similar the two amino acids are in terms of their size, electrical charge and other physical and chemical properties. If the two amino acids are similar, the substitution may not change the protein's level of activity. If they are different, however, the substitution may significantly reduce (or perhaps even increase) the level of activity of the protein.

For example, consider the apolipoprotein E (ApoE) gene, which is one of the genes that influence your risk for both heart disease and Alzheimer disease (a progressive disease where specific areas of the brain are affected and people suffer from loss of memory and other mental abilities). The most common cause of heart disease is atherosclerosis, or hardening of the arteries. Calcium, fats and cholesterol collect in blood vessels to form plaques (deposits on the vessel walls) that can trigger a heart attack or stroke. The ApoE protein works by regulating levels of certain fats in the bloodstream. High activity in the ApoE protein reduces the accumulation of these deposits, and therefore reduces the person's risk for atherosclerosis, while low activity in the ApoE protein increases the person's risk.

The ApoE gene is approximately 900 base pairs long, and has three common alleles, called E2, E3 and E4. There are two SNPs in the ApoE gene's sequence, each of which causes a single amino acid substitution (one at amino acid number 112, and the other at amino acid number 158). As Figure 5.2 illustrates, the E2 allele makes a version of the ApoE protein that has the electrically uncharged amino acid cysteine at both positions 112 and 158. In contrast, the version of the protein that is made by the E3 allele has cysteine at position112, but the positively charged amino acid arginine in position 158. The version made by the E4 allele has arginine at both positions. As we discussed in Chapter 2, substituting a positively charged amino acid (arginine) for an uncharged one (cysteine) will change the shape of the protein in that region, and will often change its level of function.

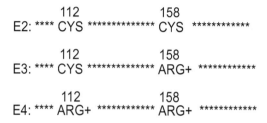

Figure 5.2. The three different versions of the ApoE protein that are made by the *ApoE* gene.

The version of the protein that is made by the E3 allele has a higher level of activity than the version that is made by the E2 and E4 alleles. The most common allele in Caucasian people of European descent is E3, which decreases the risk for atherosclerosis. Approximately 7% of Caucasian people of European descent have two copies of the E4 allele, however, and 4% have two copies of the E2 allele. Those who have these alleles have a higher risk of developing early onset heart disease than the typical person from this ethnic group has. People who possess the E4 allele also have a greater risk of developing Alzheimer disease than the typical person does.

Duplications Can Produce Extra Copies Of Genes

There are a surprising number of duplications in the typical person's DNA sequence. The duplicated stretches of DNA can be up to 1,000,000 bases long, and contain entire copies of one or more genes. If these extra copies of the gene produce protein, the person will have an excess of that protein, which can have harmful consequences.

For example, the protein CYP2D6 breaks down a number of commonly prescribed drugs. Some people have duplications in their DNA that cause them to have as many as 13 copies of the *CYP2D6* gene, rather than the two they are supposed to have. In some of these people, it appears that the extra copies of the gene are functional. These people break down several prescription drugs faster than the typical person does, and therefore need to be prescribed higher doses of these drugs than the typical person does.

The Effect Of A Deletion Or Insertion Depends On Its Size

The effect an insertion or deletion in the gene's sequence has on the protein's level of activity depends on how many bases are inserted or deleted. Recall from Chapter 2 that the ribosome reads the gene's mRNA three bases at a time, and each three-base codon directs the ribosome to add one amino acid to the protein. As Figure 5.1 illustrates, when the number of inserted or deleted bases is not a multiple of three (Figure 5.1 illustrates a single-base insertion and deletion), it alters the set of mRNA codons the ribosome reads (this is referred to as shifting the ribosome's reading frame), and causes the ribosome to chain together amino acids that do not belong in that protein. Sequence alterations that shift the ribosome's reading frame almost always cause the ribosome to make a protein that does not work.

In contrast, if the number of bases that are inserted into or deleted from the gene's sequence is a multiple of three (ex. 3, 6, 9, etc), this may cause there to be one or more amino acids inserted into or deleted from the protein. In these cases, however, because the ribosome's reading frame has not been shifted, the amino acid sequence of the protein will be normal both before and after the inserted or deleted amino acids. If the number of amino acids that gets inserted or deleted is not too high, this may not alter the level of activity in the gene's protein significantly. Most proteins have regions in which any change in the amino acid sequence will disrupt the activity of the protein, but most proteins also have regions in which substitutions or small insertions or deletions of a few amino acids will not change the protein's activity level.

Repeated Sequences Can Influence The Activity Of Genes And Proteins

Another interesting genetic variation that gets tested for in some situations involves repeated sequences in the DNA. In most places in the DNA sequence, if you read the base sequence you would see an array of As, Cs, Gs and Ts that did not form any pattern you could detect. In some genes, however there will be a portion of the gene's sequence in which a short sequence is repeated. The size of the repeated sequence varies from a single base to very long stretches of sequence. Different people will have a different number of repetitions of the repeated sequence, and the number of repetitions of the repeated sequence you have can influence the level of activity in one of your genes and/ or its protein.

For example, there is a gene called *DAT1*, whose protein helps control the function of a number of nerve pathways in your brain. There is a portion of the *DAT1* sequence in which a 40-base sequence is repeated multiple times. Most people have either 9 or 10 repetitions of the 40-base sequence (*i.e.* they have the 9-repeat or 10-repeat allele of *DAT1*). People who have the 10-repeat allele make more of the DAT1 protein than people with the 9-repeat allele do, and therefore have a higher level of activity in that protein.

Some Tests Focus On Regulatory Sequences Rather Than The Gene's Coding Sequence

Genetic tests are not necessarily restricted to analysing the gene's coding sequence and predicting changes in the amino acid content of the gene's protein. Recall from Chapter 2 that each gene has stretches of sequence that regulate the level of activity of the gene; the promoter region of the gene often contains several regulatory sequences. Because these sequences regulate the level of activity in the gene, base substitutions, duplications, insertions and deletions in these regulatory sequences may alter the amount of that protein the person has in his/her body.

For example, when a nerve cell fires, a specialised transporter protein takes the neurotransmitter that the nerve cell released back up into the nerve that released it, as a means of turning off that nerve's effect on its target nerve. One of the neurotransmitters that is used by many of your brain's nerve pathways is called serotonin (formal name = 5-hydroxytryptamine, abbreviated 5HT). The serotonin transporter protein (5HTT) helps regulate activity in a number of your brain's neural pathways. The *5HTT* gene that makes this protein has an insertion/deletion polymorphism in its promoter region. Some people have a particular 44-bp stretch of sequence in the promoter region of the *5HTT* gene (the insertion allele), while other people do not have those 44 bp (the deletion allele). Because this promoter region polymorphism influences the activity of the *5HTT* gene, and the 5HTT protein influences activity in so many of your brain's neural pathways, this polymorphism could conceivably influence many aspects of your personality and behavior.

Single-Gene Tests Versus Multiple-Gene Tests

Single-Gene Tests Are Useful When The Risk-Increasing Allele Has High Penetrance

There are a number of situations in which tests that focus on a single gene are useful. There have been a great many tests designed that can detect the gene mutations that are responsible for single-gene diseases. Because these mutations can cause the associated diseases by themselves, without needing any other genetic or nongenetic factors to contribute, testing a single gene can allow you to accurately predict whether the individual will develop that disease or not.

The situation is more complicated for multifactorial diseases, however. Most of the risk-increasing alleles that contribute to multifactorial diseases have limited **penetrance**. The penetrance of a risk-increasing allele is defined as the percentage of people who have the risk-increasing allele and also have the disease. People who have the risk-increasing allele but do not develop the disease (because they do not have the other critical genetic and/or nongenetic factors) represent examples of **nonpenetrance** of that risk-increasing allele. The mutations that cause single-gene diseases can be considered risk-increasing alleles that have 100% penetrance. Many of the risk-increasing alleles that contribute to multifactorial diseases have far less than 100% penetrance. There are some, however, whose penetrance is high enough that testing the person's status for that mutation alone can enable you to accurately predict that person's risk for developing the associated disease.

For example, some of the risk-increasing alleles in the breast cancer genes *BRCA1* and *BRCA2* have 85% penetrance, and some of the mutations in the *TP53* gene (which can contribute to several types of cancer) have greater than 90% penetrance when it comes to causing cancer. Knowing that you have one of these highly penetrant risk-increasing alleles tells you that your risk for cancer is very high. In situations such as these, a test that is focused on a single gene, and sometimes even just a single place in that gene's sequence, can provide valuable information that allows you to estimate your risk for the disease, and guides your decisions regarding the age at which you begin getting regular screenings, and how frequently you get them.

There are also a number of situations in which single-gene tests can help predict the likelihood that you will suffer a dangerous side effect after you take a particular prescription drug. There are a number of situations in which one protein plays the major role in metabolising a particular drug. In these cases, a test that focuses on the gene that makes that protein will provide information that enables the doctor to adjust the dose of the drug he/she prescribes, in order to maximise the drug's safety and effectiveness for you. For example, the enzyme NAT2 plays a major role in metabolising several commonly prescribed drugs, including hydralazine (Apresoline), which is prescribed for some people who have high blood pressure. Most people fall into one of three groups with respect to the speed with which their body metabolises hydralazine: fast metabolisers, moderate metabolisers and slow metabolisers. If you know which alleles the individual has at a few important sites in the *NAT2* sequence, you can predict the speed at which his/her body will metabolise hydralazine, and prescribe the dose that will be as safe and effective as possible for that person.

Multi-Gene Test Panels Will Be Powerful Diagnostic Tools And Predictors Of Risk

There are a number of tests that are being developed in which the sequences of several genes are analysed simultaneously. These tests provide advantages both in cases of single-gene diseases and in cases of multifactorial diseases as well.

Some single-gene diseases may be due to a mutation in one of several genes. If the required genetic tests are expensive, it is often the best strategy to test the genes one at a time, beginning with the gene that has been reported to be mutated most frequently in the current patient's ethnic group. As the cost of genetic testing declines, however, it will become more common to use a multi-gene test panel to quickly determine the cause of that person's disease. In some cases, determining which gene contains the mutation that caused the disease may help the doctor decide which of several alternative treatments will be most effective for that particular patient.

Multi-gene tests are essential if you want to predict someone's risk for a multifactorial disease. For most multifactorial diseases, there are many risk-increasing gene alleles that could possibly be present in any person who has that disease. Different people who have the same disease will have different combinations of the critical genetic (and nongenetic) factors. In order to determine which risk-increasing alleles one individual has for the disease of interest as quickly as possible, you need a test panel that is capable of detecting all the risk-increasing alleles that might contribute to that disease.

Multi-gene testing panels are essential for determining the causes of multifactorial diseases because your metabolism is organised into metabolic pathways. Each metabolic pathway is a series of chemical reactions that together accomplish some metabolic goal (ex. harvesting energy from stored fat). A metabolic pathway may be simple, and consist of only a few different reactions, or highly complex, and include dozens of different reactions. In most cases, each reaction in the pathway is run by a different protein (the proteins that run your body's chemical reactions are called enzymes). Because so many proteins work together in each pathway, if you have an unusually high or low level of activity in one protein, that will usually not alter the level of activity in that metabolic pathway significantly. If someone has two or more risk-increasing alleles that affect the activity of multiple proteins that work together in the same metabolic pathway, however, the effects of these genetic factors may multiply each other, or even interact more dramatically than that.

There are two implications that stem from this. The first is that any single risk-increasing allele will have low penetrance, because you will not develop the disease unless you also possess one or more additional genetic (and perhaps also nongenetic) factors. The second is that, in order to develop a test that predicts your risk for most multifactorial diseases, you need to design a test that gives you information about the activity levels of dozens, even hundreds, of proteins.

Microarrays Enable Many Genes To Be Tested At Once

One of the technologies that enables the testing laboratory to obtain information about a great many genes at once involves the use of **microarrays**, or "**gene chips**." The most commonly used microarrays are made from glass slides, onto which millions of pieces of synthetic DNA[1] (called probes) are applied in tiny micro-spots (Figures 5.3 and 5.4). These probes will bind to human DNA (a process usually referred to as **hybridisation**), following the complementary base pair rule we discussed in Chapter 2 (A bases bind to T bases, C bases bind to G bases). Because each probe contains a different sequence of bases, each probe will only bind to a specific sequence in the DNA that is being tested.

Figure 5.3 illustrates the basic principle behind these hybridisation-based microarray assays. In order to determine the person's sequence for a particular SNP, because there are four possible sequences, or alleles, of that SNP (there could be either an A, C, G or T there), you need four probes[2]. Each probe will have a sequence that is designed to hybridise with only one of the four possible alleles of that SNP.

The DNA undergoes a special preparation procedure, including a process that makes it fluoresce (glow) when you shine a particular color light on it. The genetic analyst lets the specially prepared DNA sit on the microarray, to enable the person's DNA to bind to the probes whose sequences are complementary to the DNA's sequence. The microarray is then washed to remove any extra DNA, whereupon the microarray is put under the appropriate color light, and a computerised system reports which probes have bound to the DNA. This tells the analyst which alleles the individual has at the SNP that is being tested (Figure 5.4).

---

[1]   Genetics equipment companies sell several versions of a machine that can synthesise short pieces of DNA containing whatever base sequence the researcher wants.

[2]   In many cases, only two alleles of the SNP have ever been observed; nobody has ever reported finding one of the other two bases in any of the sequences they have analysed. In these cases, the array may only include probes that bind to the two previously-reported alleles.

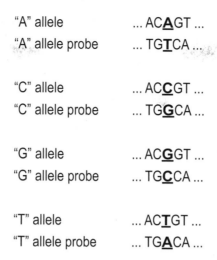

"A" allele	... AC**A**GT ...
"A" allele probe	... TG**T**CA ...
"C" allele	... AC**C**GT ...
"C" allele probe	... TG**G**CA ...
"G" allele	... AC**G**GT ...
"G" allele probe	... TG**C**CA ...
"T" allele	... AC**T**GT ...
"T" allele probe	... TG**A**CA ...

Figure 5.3. The four different sequences you might find at a SNP, and the probe sequences that would bind to them.

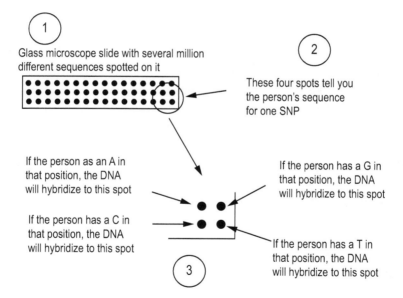

Figure 5.4. Illustration of the principle behind microarray-based hybridisation assays.

The most recent versions of microarrays can fit 2.7 million different probes on them. That means that a single microarray can provide information about hundreds of thousands, even millions, of different gene polymorphisms in one assay. Given the tremendous capacity of a microarray, there will be few diseases for which researchers cannot design a microarray that tests polymorphisms from all the critical genes (once they determine which genes are the critical ones).

Whole-Genome Screens Provide Information About A Lot Of Genes At Once

At present, the most extensive version of the multi-gene test panel that has been developed is the whole-genome SNP screen. Whole-genome SNP screening involves testing the individual's DNA to determine which base he/she has for approximately 1 million (1,000,000) SNPs that are distributed throughout the DNA sequence. These whole-genome SNP screens are offered directly to consumers by several genetic testing companies. Given the large number of SNPs that can be tested in one of these whole-genome SNP screens, these tests can yield a huge amount of information. They can provide information about your risk for many diseases or drug responses, your personal characteristics and your ancestry.

Microarrays Can Also Detect Copy Number Variations

One of the more surprising discoveries that have recently been reported about human DNA is that there are a great many **copy number variations** in the typical person's DNA. It is generally assumed that we have two copies of every gene (except for males' X and Y chromosome genes). It has recently become apparent, however, that the typical person has many deletions, duplications and insertions in his/her DNA sequence. Some of these deleted/duplicated/inserted stretches of DNA are 1,000,000 bp long; many of them are large enough to contain one or more genes. This results in many people having either one (through deletion) or three or more (from duplication or insertion) copies of some of their genes. Microarrays can be used to determine how many copies of the gene of interest the person has.

One example of this involves a gene called CYP2D6, whose protein metabolises a large number of commonly prescribed drugs. Some people have duplications that give them extra copies of the CYP2D6 gene (some have 13 copies of the gene!). Researchers are not certain whether all those extra copies of CYP2D6 are active, but it seems that at least some of them are active in some people, because some of the people who have extra copies of CYP2D6 metabolise CYP2D6's target drugs more rapidly than most other people do. These individuals need to be prescribed higher doses of any drugs that the CYP2D6 protein metabolises, because they often will not get any benefit from the typical dose.

SEQUENCING ALLOWS YOU TO DETECT ALL THE SEQUENCE VARIANTS IN A GENE

No matter how many different SNPs you include in a whole-genome SNP screen, these tests all suffer from two limitations: they only look at one or a few sites in any given gene, and they only look for sequence variants that have been reported before. Sequencing overcomes these two limitations: it provides information about every base in the gene's sequence, and it enables the analyst to detect all the variants you possess in that gene's sequence, including ones that have not been reported in the literature before.

Once the cost of sequencing DNA declines to a certain level, sequencing will represent the best combination of information and cost, and will be used increasingly more frequently in personalised medicine tests. A person's DNA sequence could conceivably be determined using the blood sample that is taken from every newborn shortly after birth. These data could be stored in databases that are linked to one's electronic medical record, so that this information can be used by you and your health care team to better estimate your risk for specific diseases and choose the safest and most effective treatments for you when you do get sick.

THE MOST USEFUL TESTS WILL COMBINE GENETIC FACTORS, NONGENETIC FACTORS AND CLINICAL INFORMATION: THE WARFARIN (COUMADIN) EXAMPLE

In order to produce tests that will estimate the person's risk for a disease or drug response most accurately, it will usually be necessary to combine information about genetic factors and nongenetic factors with personal information and clinical data such as blood sugar level or blood pressure. Genomic researchers are trying to develop formulas that combine each of the relevant factors in a way that gives the factors that are most important the most weight, and counts the others a little less heavily (you may see these types of formulas referred to as algorithms). In fact, determining exactly how to combine the relevant factors into a predictive formula is one of the biggest challenges facing researchers who are trying to develop these formulas.

For example, let's consider one formula that has been suggested for calculating the person's dose of the blood thinner warfarin (Coumadin). Warfarin has a narrow **therapeutic window**; this means that there is a relatively small difference between an effective dose of the drug and a dangerously high dose of the drug. With a blood thinner like warfarin, you've got to get the dose just right. Too little, and the patient risks blood clots, which can be fatal. Too much, and the blood is too thin; the patient risks internal bleeding.

There are four genes whose proteins' levels of activity influence the way your body will respond to warfarin. In addition to information about your sequence for these four genes, one formula for calculating a person's dose of warfarin also considers the number of doses of warfarin you have already had, your age, sex, ethnicity, height and weight, whether you smoke, have liver disease, why exactly you are being prescribed warfarin, and whether you are taking certain other drugs.

It will take a little time for researchers to develop extremely accurate formulas for many situations, because we still have not identified the critical genetic and nongenetic factors that influence many diseases/drug reactions. In addition, it will require large research studies, with many subjects in them, before researchers know exactly how to combine the critical factors into their respective formulas. As the declining cost of whole-genome sequencing and microarray analyses allows researchers to use these technologies for more of their studies, however, the pace at which researchers gather new information that can be used to refine these predictive formulas will go from its already impressive pace to a staggering one.

The Field Will Progress Slowly But Surely

At this point, there are only a few fields of medicine in which personalised medicine tests are making a significant impact. These examples have proven the principles behind personalised medicine, however, and have demonstrated that personalised medicine tests can improve the safety and effectiveness of treatments, as well as reduce the cost of health care. The early research in this field has had its share of problems, but a great many important lessons have been learned, and programs are in place to insure that the tests that are being developed today will truly help your doctor estimate your risk for diseases or choose the right treatment for you.

As researchers discover more about the genetic and nongenetic factors that influence your risk for disease or response to drugs, the scope of personalised medicine tests will grow. The most useful tests will include genetic, nongenetic, family history, personal and clinical information. In addition, these formulas will combine these different pieces of information in a manner that takes into account how strongly each one influences the person's risk for the disease in question. Although none of the tests that are available today combine all these diverse types of information, it is only a matter of time before enough is known about the factors that contribute to diseases, and the means by which they interact, to develop these comprehensive tests.

The list of personalised medicine tests that are available will continue to grow rapidly in the near future; no book can hope to provide current information. The National

Institute of Health maintains the GeneTests website (http://www.ncbi.nlm.nih.gov/sites/GeneTests/), which provides the most comprehensive and current listing of personalised medicine tests that are available. The website is written for doctors, so there may be some things that are too technical for the lay person to understand, but you may want to be sure your doctor knows about it. He/she can search the website by using a specific disease as a search term, and find out what the current status of personalised medicine is for any given disease.

CHAPTER SUMMARY

- Personalised medicine tests provide many benefits. They enable your doctor to estimate your risk for specific diseases, diagnose diseases more accurately and design a treatment plan that will be as safe and effective for you as possible. They can also screen prospective parents for recessive mutations, and determine whether or not a fetus has inherited a parent's mutation.

- Genetic tests can detect a variety of abnormalities in the DNA sequence, including base substitutions, duplications, insertions, deletions, repeated sequence length polymorphisms, extra or missing copies of a gene, and changes in regulatory sequences that will affect the level of activity in a gene.

- While single-gene tests can be useful in many situations, it is often beneficial to test multiple genes for sequence variations, especially in the case of multifactorial diseases. Microarrays enable one to test for hundreds of thousands of DNA sequence variations at once, and whole-genome sequencing allows one to see all the sequence variations a person has.

- The most useful personalised medicine tests will combine information about genetic factors, nongenetic factors, personal medical history, family medical history and other personal information.

CHAPTER 6

MAKING THE DECISION WHETHER OR NOT TO HAVE GENETIC TESTING, AND INTERPRETING THE RESULTS OF TESTS YOU CHOOSE TO HAVE PERFORMED

Making The Decision Whether Or Not To Have Genetic Testing

Personalised Medicine Encourages You To Take A More Active Role In Maintaining Your Health

Personalised medicine aims to individualise health care, rather than having doctors treat everyone with a particular disease with the same treatment plan. The personalised medicine tests of the future will combine information about your personal health history, family history, age, gene sequences, medical information such as blood sugar or cholesterol level, diet, environment and lifestyle. By assessing this information for each individual patient, doctors will be better able to predict the individual's risk for specific diseases, as well as diagnose diseases more confidently. In addition, in some cases this information will enable your doctor to design the safest and most effective treatment plan for you when you get sick.

Personalised medicine will not just enable your doctor to do his/her job better; it will help you maintain your own health more effectively. Genetic and nongenetic factors interact to influence our risks for many of the most common diseases. Thus, if you know the diseases for which you have the greatest genetic risk, you may be able to minimise your exposure to some of the nongenetic factors that increase your risk of developing that disease. In some cases, personalised medicine tests may enable you to avoid developing a specific disease entirely. In other cases, the information may allow you to delay the onset of the disease, or reduce the severity of the disease.

Personalised medicine has been called P4™ Medicine: Predictive, Preventive, Personalised, and Participatory Medicine. The term "participatory" refers to the fact that this new approach to medicine includes having people play a more active role in maintaining their own health and making decisions regarding their medical care than they usually do. By allowing each of us to be informed about our genetic and nongenetic risks, personalised medicine testing can empower us to make changes that might impact our long-term health in positive ways. It requires a certain amount of discipline to make many of these changes, however, and people must motivate themselves to take this active role in maintaining their own health.

Genetic Testing Can Have A Significant Psychological And Emotional Impact

Different people have different reasons for wanting genetic testing. Some people are interested in obtaining information about physical traits, or their ancestry, while others want genetic testing for health-related reasons. Anyone who is considering having genetic testing performed must understand exactly what information is going to be provided by the test. This is particularly true if you have a whole-genome SNP screen or whole-genome sequencing performed; these tests may provide information you were not expecting. For example, someone who had a whole-genome analysis performed wanting information about physical traits or ancestry may be taken by surprise when he/she learns that he/she possesses a risk-increasing allele for cancer or sudden cardiac death. Whole-genome sequencing will potentially provide information about a great many diseases. There may be things a person can do to reduce his/her risk for some of these diseases, but for others, there may be nothing the person can do. These tests might also reveal information about sensitive issues, such as psychiatric disorders, behavior traits and non-paternity.

It is particularly difficult to make the decision whether or not to have genetic testing performed when the test may reveal that you have an increased risk for a condition for which there is currently no effective treatment or cure (such as Alzheimer disease). A genetic test that reveals that you have a risk-increasing gene allele that has high penetrance tells you that you have a very good chance of developing that disease. Different people will face this kind of information with different attitudes. Some people will want to know that they possess the risk-increasing allele, feeling that it will enable them to prepare for the future more effectively. Others will not want to know this information, because it will cause them to focus too much on the fact that they are going to develop the disease. Some people may worry that the resultant depression and anxiety will reduce the quality of their life during the healthy period they expect to have before the disease develops.

The different attitudes that different people have regarding genetic testing for uncurable diseases have been most clearly illustrated in the case of Huntington's disease

(HD). This is a progressive disease in which your nervous system degenerates and you progressively lose many of your mental abilities and your physical coordination. Huntington's disease is caused by an autosomal dominant mutation in the *huntingtin* gene. If one of your parents is affected with Huntington's disease, you have a 50% probability of developing the disease yourself.

Because the symptoms of HD usually begin developing when the person is in their 30s-40s, some people who have a parent with HD may seek testing to see if they are at risk or not. If you learn that you have inherited the HD mutation from your affected parent, not only does this tell you that you can expect to develop HD, but it also tells you that you have a 50% probability of passing the mutation down to any one of your children. If you learn that you do not possess the mutation, however, you know that your risk for HD is very low--equal to the typical person's risk.

Finding out that you did not inherit the HD mutation from your affected parent can lead to a wide range of emotions. While you will certainly feel a certain amount of relief at hearing the news, some people may also feel survivor's guilt because they were spared the disease other family members are suffering from. Because of the potential emotional impact associated with genetic testing, some people whose parents have HD choose not to learn whether they also possess the parent's mutation. Interestingly, this group of people includes one of the researchers on the team that discovered that mutations in the *huntingtin* gene cause HD[1] and developed the genetic test for HD.

Genetic Counselors Help You Determine If A Genetic Test Is Right For You

Genetic counselors provide many different services related to genetic, genomic and personalised medicine testing. Some genetic counselors specialise in a particular area of medicine, such as cardiovascular (heart) disease, while others provide genetic counseling for a range of conditions.

During a typical meeting with a genetic counselor, the counselor will collect a complete family history, ask a number of questions about your diet, environment and lifestyle, and take the time to answer any questions you have. The counselor will provide an estimate of your risk for specific diseases, and explain the potential risks and benefits associated with the genetic/genomic tests that are available to you. The genetic counselor will also discuss any issues identified in your personal and family medical history that may indicate that you have an increased risk for any rare genetic diseases. If genetic/genomic testing is done, he/she will help you interpret the results of

---

[1]   Dr. Nancy Wexler, a professor at Columbia University

the tests you had performed. A genetic counselor can help educate you about all aspects of genetic diseases and genetic/genomic testing, and explain how the information from your genetic/genomic tests must be combined with information about your family medical history and your exposure to nongenetic factors in order to appreciate its significance to your health and medical care. If the genetic/genomic testing suggests that your risk for a specific disease is higher or lower than that which is predicted from your family medical history, the counselor will discuss that, and resolve the conflict if possible. The counselor will also try to anticipate any ways in which the significance of your test results may change, or recommendations for your health care may change, as new discoveries are made.

The genetic counselor will discuss a number of health-related issues, including the current recommendations and guidelines regarding screening procedures such as mammograms, blood sugar testing or blood pressure monitoring. In addition, the counselor will also discuss the implications that any genetic/genomic tests that were performed have for your family members. Finally, one of the counselor's most important roles is to offer support and counseling to address the emotional and family issues that may arise when a genetic condition is identified in a family, or when a client is found to have an increased risk for a particular disease. Counselors are aware that, when faced with the news that they have a specific level of risk for a given disease, different people will react differently. Any individual person's emotional response to the news will depend on his/her age, values and life circumstances. Genetic counselors can not only provide you with the support, education, consultation and guidance you need, but they can also provide these services for your family members, and work with your health care providers to be sure you get the maximum benefit from your genetic/genomic tests.

Recently Passed Laws Insure Your Privacy

One of the concerns many people have when they consider having genetic testing performed is protection of their personal genetic information. People are concerned that insurance companies or employers might discriminate against them, or that the companies that advertise their services directly to consumers (direct-to-consumer, or DTC companies) might sell their customers' genomic data to pharmaceutical companies or other businesses. Even the strongest supporter of genetic testing must agree that this is a concern.

Fortunately, the Genetic Insurance Nondiscrimination Act (GINA) of 2008 provides some strong safeguards against using people's genetic information to deny them insurance policies or jobs based on their predicted long-term health status. In addition, the National Institutes of Health has implemented strict controls to protect the privacy of your genetic information, and many DTC testing laboratories also protect the data they have stored. These measures do not completely allay all concerns. For example, GINA does not specify all the relevant regulations or the penalties for illegally accessing people's genetic information. There will no doubt be further changes made to GINA, or other laws passed to protect the privacy of people's genetic data. There are several websites you can visit to get information about the current state of GINA. One is the Genetics and Public policy center at Johns Hopkins University, at http://www.dnapolicy.org/gina/gina.overview.html. The site has a complete overview of the Act, plus a page with answers to frequently asked questions.

THE IDEAL GENETIC TEST REPORT SHOULD INCLUDE SPECIFIC INFORMATION ABOUT YOUR RISK-INCREASING AND RISK-DECREASING ALLELES: WE ARE NOT THERE YET

At this time, there is no standard format for reporting the results of genetic tests; different laboratories will provide different specific types of information in their reports. Unfortunately, few reports provide the kind of detailed information that enables you to interpret the full significance of the test result. In some cases, the report omits information that could have been provided, but in other cases we still do not know enough about certain sequence variants to determine whether they will change the level of activity in any of your proteins (discussed in more detail below). In addition, there is still a lot we do not know about how the information from genetic/genomic tests must be combined with information about nongenetic risk factors, medical data such as blood sugar level, and family history data in order to produce the most accurate estimate possible of your risk for a specific disease.

Knowing The Penetrance Of A Risk-Increasing Allele Helps You Understand Its Significance

There are a number of things you might want to know about the risk-increasing alleles you possess. One of the most important pieces of information you would want to know is the degree of **penetrance** for any risk-increasing alleles that are found. Penetrance is defined as the percentage of people who have the gene variant in question and also develop the disease. The risk-increasing alleles that contribute to multifactorial diseases usually have less than 100% penetrance, because it usually requires the person to have one or more additional risk-increasing gene alleles, or exposure to some critical nongenetic factors, in order to develop the disease. There is always some percentage of people who have any given risk-increasing gene allele who never develop the disease (these people represent cases of nonpenetrance of the risk-increasing allele). These people may not have the other critical gene variations, they may not have been exposed to the critical nongenetic factors, or they may also have one or more risk-reducing gene alleles (Figure 6.1). Reporting the penetrance of a risk-increasing allele gives the person an idea of just how strongly that single genetic factor influences his/her risk for the disease in question.

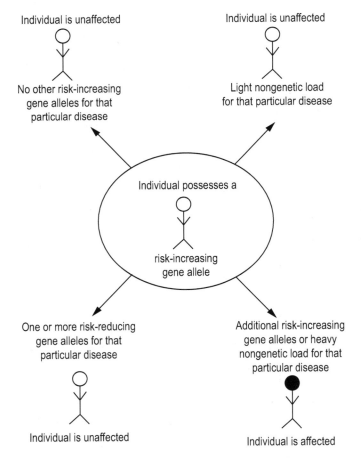

Figure 6.1. There are a number of reasons why an individual may have the risk-increasing allele for a gene, but not have the disease. These cases are examples of nonpenetrance of the risk-increasing allele.

Another way to understand just how significantly a given risk-increasing allele elevates your risk for a disease is to know the **relative risk** that is associated with that particular allele. Relative risk is a simple concept. Someone who possesses a risk-increasing allele that has a relative risk of 2.0 is twice as likely as the typical person to develop the disease that has been associated with that allele, while someone who possesses a risk-increasing allele with a relative risk of 3.0 is three times as likely as the typical person to develop the disease that has been associated with that allele. For example, there is a cluster of SNPs on chromosome 9, one or more of which is believed to influence people's risk for heart disease. One of the risk-increasing alleles is the C allele of a SNP that is called rs1333049. Possessing one copy of the C allele gives you a relative risk of 1.3 for coronary artery disease, while possessing two copies of the C allele of rs1333049 gives you a relative risk of 1.7.

In most cases, your risk for developing the disease in question can be estimated simply by taking the population risk for the disease in question (the risk for the "typical" person of your age, sex and ethnicity), and multiplying it by the relative risk that is assigned to the risk-increasing allele that you possess. This is not ideal, because it gives you an estimate based on population data, whereas your best estimate will only be obtained by including your personal family history and nongenetic factor information as well. It does, however, give you an impression of how much having that risk-increasing allele influences your risk of developing the disease.

Ideally, in order to produce an accurate estimate of the probability that you will develop the disease in question, you would want someone to combine the results of the genetic test (including risk-reducing alleles as well as risk-increasing alleles) with family history, nongenetic and personal data. These estimates should always include a timeframe. For example, you may be told that you have a 1 in 25 chance of developing a specific disease before you are 70, or during your entire life. In many cases, however, we do not yet know enough about the effects of that risk-increasing allele, or the factors with which it interacts, to provide accurate timeframe estimates.

After reading the previous chapters, you are aware that the issues that arise when someone possesses a risk-increasing allele differ from one case to another, depending on the specific gene, allele, disease and person involved. Although some of the commercial testing companies provide educational materials on their websites that can help you understand the test results, it is often essential to seek help from a genetic counselor in order to understand all the implications of your test results and have all your questions answered.

The Relative Risk Tells You How Much Protection You Get From A Risk-Reducing Allele

In addition to risk-increasing alleles, the report may state that you also have one or more gene alleles that reduce your risk for a specific disease. In cases such as these, the best way to assess the degree of protection you get from possessing that allele is to know the relative risk that is associated with that allele. Because the relative risk compares your risk to that of the typical person, risk-increasing alleles have relative risks greater than 1.0, while risk-reducing alleles will have relative risks that are less than 1.0. This is probably the best way to explain the degree of protection you get from that allele, but unfortunately, there are many cases in which we still do not know enough about the effects of risk-reducing alleles to provide an accurate relative risk estimate.

The Absence Of A Disease-Causing Mutation Does Not Mean You Have Zero Risk

People who have a parent who possesses a gene mutation that causes a specific single-gene disease often want to have genetic testing performed in order to determine if they have inherited their parent's mutation. If the report states that you did not inherit the mutation, you should not interpret this as indicating that you have zero risk for that disease. When the family's mutation is known, these tests often focus only on that site in the gene. If that site has a normal sequence, you may still have a mutation elsewhere in that gene, a mutation in another gene that can cause the disease, or you may be exposed to nongenetic factors that increase your risk for that disease. If the report states that you did not inherit the mutation that your parent had, you should interpret that as stating that your risk for the disease is the same as the typical person's risk, which is always greater than zero.

At Present, Risk Estimates Are Not Very Specific

It would be ideal if personalised medicine tests could give people specific numerical estimates of their risks of developing specific diseases. This is already possible for the mutations that cause single-gene diseases and some of the risk-increasing alleles that contribute to multifactorial diseases, but for many of the gene alleles that increase your risk for multifactorial diseases, we still do not know enough to provide a specific numerical estimate of your risk. Instead, your risk is usually stated as low, medium or high compared to the typical person's risk for that disease. In general, you can conceptualise the interaction between genetic and nongenetic factors as it is portrayed in Table 6-1. If you have favorable genetic and nongenetic factors, your risk for the disease is low. If you have risk-increasing genetic or nongenetic factors, your risk will be medium. If you have unfavorable genetic and nongenetic factors, your risk will be high.

Table 6-1. Categories Of Risk As They Are Usually Reported

	Favorable Genetic Factors	Unfavorable Genetic Factors
Favorable Nongenetic Factors	Low risk	Medium Risk
Unfavorable Nongenetic Factors	Medium Risk	High Risk

INTERPRETATION ISN'T ALWAYS EASY; THE CURRENTLY AVAILABLE TESTS HAVE SOME IMPORTANT LIMITATIONS

There Is A Surprising Amount Of Genetic Variation In Healthy People

As we discussed in Chapter 1, there appears to be a great deal of variation in the "normal" human DNA sequence; the typical person's DNA has a surprising number of SNPs, insertions, deletions and other rearrangements compared to the reference human DNA sequence. Some of these variants are not predicted to have any effect on their protein's activity level, but some of them are predicted to exert a significant effect on the protein's activity.

One of the most interesting discoveries researchers have recently made about human DNA is that a surprising number of healthy people have less than, or more than, the two copies of each gene that we assume they have[2]. Deletions and duplications of portions of the DNA are known to cause many different developmental abnormalities. For example, many people who have Duchenne muscular dystrophy have deletions on their X chromosome, while people who have Down syndrome often have an extra copy of the entire chromosome 21. It was surprising, however, to discover that so many healthy people have deletions and duplications that change the number of copies they have of one or more genes. As described below, a significant minority of people have extra copies of some of the *CYP450* genes, whose proteins metabolise many prescription and nonprescription drugs. Some of these people need to be given higher doses of those drugs, because their bodies break the drug down so quickly that the typical dose does not build up enough of a concentration in their bodies to be effective.

The effects of these genetic variations are not restricted to prescription drugs or diseases. They can affect our responses to over-the-counter drugs, as well as things we

---

[2] We expect everyone to have two copies of each gene, except males, who have one copy of each of their X and Y chromosome genes.

consume that we don't often consider drugs. For example, the direct-to-consumer tests often test the individual's status for the *CYP1A2* gene, which makes one of the many members of the huge family of CYP450 proteins. The CYP1A2 protein metabolises caffeine; possessing one or more low-activity alleles of *CYP1A2* increases the risk of heart attack for people who drink large amounts of coffee. Your status for the *CYP1A2* gene may also affect how well you tolerate a lack of coffee if you are accustomed to drinking it regularly but are unable to get access to some.

The enormous level of variability that exists in the human genome was illustrated in an article that described the sequencing of Dr. James Lupski's genome (http://content. nejm.org/cgi/content/full/NEJMoa0908094). Dr. Lupski is a genetic researcher who suffers from a somewhat rare single-gene disease known as Charcot-Marie Tooth (CMT) syndrome, a neurological condition that results in muscle weakness and wasting. Dr. Lupski has been searching for the genetic cause of his disease for decades, and became one of the first people in the world to have their genome fully sequenced. The sequencing of Dr. Lupski's entire DNA molecule helped genomic researchers identify the gene mutation that caused him to have CMT. In addition, however, it illustrated just how difficult it is to identify the gene variants that contribute to disease, even when you have the entire sequence of the individual's DNA to work with.

Charcot-Marie Tooth disease is a single-gene disease; there are several different versions of CMT, each of which is caused by a mutation in a different gene. Because it is a single-gene disease, it is possible to pinpoint a single gene mutation as the sole cause of that individual's disease. None of this work is easy, but trying to identify the sole cause of a single-gene disease is considerably easier than trying to identify all the genetic and nongenetic factors that influence susceptibility to most multifactorial diseases. When they analysed Dr. Lupski's DNA sequence, researchers were surprised to discover that Dr. Lupski's DNA sequence contained thousands of sequence variants that could significantly influence the level of activity in their respective genes' proteins. Most shockingly, Dr. Lupski's genome also contained 121 instances in which there was a STOP codon in the sequence of a gene that was expected to be actively making its protein. Recall from Chapter 2 that a STOP codon causes the cell to stop adding amino acids to the growing protein. The protein ends right there, and is missing whichever amino acids were supposed to be added on after that point. This often results in the protein being unable to function, and mutations that create premature STOP codons are the cause of many single-gene diseases.

One of those mutations that caused a premature STOP codon to appear in the gene's sequence was located in one of the genes that had already been reported to be mutated in several other people who have CMT. This appears to be the gene mutation that caused Dr. Lupski to have CMT. If it was not for the fact that this gene had already been identified as a gene that could be involved in CMT, however, it would have been very difficult to be certain that particular gene variant was the cause of Dr. Lupski's CMT. In addition to that mutation, there were 120 other sequence variations that were predicted to causes premature STOP codons in their gene's sequence, and thousands of others that might have disrupted their protein's function as well. We have all heard expressions that refer to how difficult it is to find a needle in a haystack. The task of identifying the gene mutation that caused Dr. Lupski's CMT was more a matter of trying to figure out which of the 121 needles you found in the haystack was the one needle you were looking for. Dr. Lupski does not have any other obvious medical diseases, so it appears that these other 120 STOP codon mutations do not have any significant effect on Dr. Lupski's health. They are probably some of the factors that give Dr. Lupski his unique combination of physical traits, emotional makeup, and other characteristics that make us all unique individuals, but they do not seem to cause any specific diseases.

The fact that Dr. Lupski does not have any genetic diseases other than CMT does not mean that these other variations that were found in his DNA sequence have no significance. Recall from Chapter 3 that many gene mutations are recessive mutations, and both copies of that gene must have the mutation in order for the individual to develop the disease. These predicted STOP codon mutations, and these insertions and deletions that were seen in Dr. Lupski's DNA, may all be recessive mutations that could cause a single-gene disease if they were present in both copies of the gene. Some of these recessive diseases can be very serious, even lethal, so findings such as these can influence not only that person's decisions about having children, but those of his family members as well. Until researchers have had time to analyse the effects of these genetic variations on health, many of the sequence variations that genetic tests find will be of unknown significance, and interpreting their significance may require testing family members.

One of the important limitations of DNA sequencing is that, if the test finds that the person has two variations in the gene's sequence, standard sequencing techniques cannot determine whether both variations occur in the same copy of the gene, or one variation occurs in each of the person's two copies of the gene. This can be an important determinant of the specific effect these sequence variations will have on the person's health. Having two mutations in the same copy of the gene will probably render that gene unable to produce a working protein, but will leave the other copy of the gene functional. In contrast, having one mutation in each of the two copies of that gene may render both copies of the gene unable to produce a functional protein.

Another important limitation of genetic testing lies in the fact that there is no central database to which researchers can turn to integrate their new discoveries with previous discoveries in the same area. At present, researchers often need to scan multiple sources of information to find everything they need to know about a specific mutation or a specific disease. Putting all the information together into one place will require the cooperative efforts of genetic counselors, medical geneticists, researchers and computer analysts. In addition, we can only interpret the findings of a test from the perspective of what we know today. In an ideal situation, as researchers discover new information about the significance of specific gene variants and the way our genetic and nongenetic factors interact, this information would be added to the existing knowledge base.

These issues raise some important questions. As new discoveries are made, we also need to find clearer ways to convey this information to people. There is also the question of who will pay the cost, not only of the testing, but of the process that is required to interpret the results of the test as well as possible.

It Isn't Always Easy To Tell What Effect A Sequence Variation Has On The Protein's Activity

Whole-genome sequencing and whole-genome SNP screens provide a tremendous amount of information, but the interpretation of the data is not always as clear-cut as you would like it to be. For example, recall from the discussion in Chapter 2 that some sequence variations cause one amino acid to be substituted for another in the protein. If the amino acids are very similar to each other with respect to their electrical charge, size and other critical properties, the amino acid substitution will probably have no impact on the protein's activity. Conversely, if the two amino acids are very different from each other, the substitution will probably have a significant effect on the activity of the protein. If, on the other hand, the two amino acids are moderately different from each other in size and charge, it may be difficult to determine exactly what impact this sequence variant will have on the activity of the protein without having someone directly study the effect of that sequence variant on the protein in a laboratory.

In addition, as we discussed in Chapter 2, each gene has a promoter region and other sequences that regulate the level of activity in the gene. Sequence variations in these regulatory sequences always have the potential to change the amount of protein the gene is making. Some authorities estimate that sequence variations in these regulatory sequences account for more of the variability in our proteins' activities than sequence variations in our genes' coding sequences do. At the present time, however, for most genes, we do not know which specific bases in the promoter region are the critical ones. It is often difficult, therefore, to determine the effect a change in sequence of the promoter region of a gene will have on the gene's level of activity.

In addition to the challenge of determining exactly which sequence variations affect the activity of their genes' proteins, researchers also face the enormous challenge of determining whether certain variants affect the protein's activity as significantly as others do. In order to develop the most useful tests possible, it is not only necessary to figure out what the important genetic factors are, but it is also necessary to figure out whether to give each factor equal weight when you combine them into a formula for calculating the person's risk.

For example, imagine there is a gene with two SNPs that influence the level of activity in the gene's protein. For SNP number 1, the risk-increasing allele completely abolishes the activity of its gene's protein, while the risk-increasing allele of SNP number 2 only reduces the level of activity in the protein by 15%. If you were to combine information from both these SNPs into a formula that was intended to calculate the person's risk for the associated disease, your formula should be constructed in a way that allows possessing one risk-increasing allele for SNP number 1 to increase the final estimate of your risk to a greater degree than possessing one risk-increasing allele in SNP number 2. In addition, the formula would need to include any risk-reducing alleles that were present in that gene, and account for the degree to which they were capable of counteracting the effects of the risk-increasing alleles.

Many Risk-Increasing SNP Alleles Only Increase Your Risk By A Small Amount

While it would be ideal to design a SNP screen that contained one or more SNPs from each gene, and only use SNPs that directly affected the activity of the protein their gene produced, it has been impossible for the early efforts at whole-genome SNP screening to take this approach. There are many genes that don't seem to have one SNP, or any other kind of variant, that exerts a significantly greater influence over the activity level of the gene's protein than the other SNPs do. Instead, it appears that many genes have several SNPs (or other variants) that each exert a small influence over the protein's activity level.

The fact that many proteins' activities appear to be influenced by several polymorphisms in the gene that makes that protein has several implications for genetic testing. For one, when a protein's activity level is influenced by several polymorphisms, each with a relatively small effect, you need to assess the status of several polymorphisms in that gene in order to determine the activity level of that protein in that person. Before you can do that, however, you must identify the critical polymorphisms. This is especially challenging for the polymorphisms that only exert small effects on the gene's protein. You have to study an especially large group of people in order to identify those variants and determine how large their effects are on a person's risk for that disease.

When each individual risk-increasing allele only influences your risk by a small amount, it is easy to attach more significance to possessing a risk-increasing allele than is appropriate. For most of the risk-increasing alleles we know of, learning that you possess that risk-increasing allele does not change much about your plan for maintaining your health. For example, imagine a disease for which the typical person's overall lifetime risk for developing the disease is 20%. Imagine further that you possess a risk-increasing allele that increases your risk for the disease by 20% compared to the typical person's. This means that, while the typical person who does not possess the risk-increasing allele has a 20% probability of developing that disease in his/her lifetime, the person with the risk-increasing allele has a 24% overall risk for developing the disease in his/her lifetime (20% of 20% is 4%, so adding the extra 4% onto the typical person's risk of 20% gives you 24%). Knowing that your risk just increased from 20% to 24% is probably not going to change your health-related habits, or your doctor's advice about medical treatments, diet, environment or lifestyle. Your risk will probably still be well below the level of risk at which people are recommended to take special measures such as earlier or more frequent screening/monitoring (Figure 6.2).

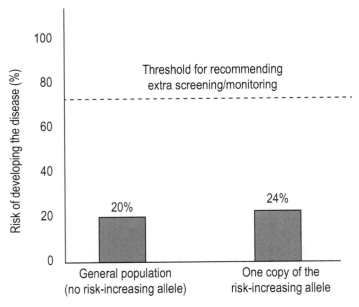

Figure 6.2. Hypothetical example illustrating how most risk-increasing alleles do not influence your risk for a disease enough to change the plan for your health care.

The SNPs Used In SNP Screens Don't Always Provide Direct, Reliable Information

The whole-genome SNP screen is supposed to provide information about the activity level in all your proteins. In an ideal situation, the test would include one or more SNPs from each of your genes, and each of these SNPs would significantly affect the activity of the protein its gene produced. Knowing which allele of a SNP the person possessed would tell you directly what level of activity that person had for that gene's protein.

Unfortunately, however, many of the SNPs that are assessed in these whole-genome SNP screens do not directly influence the activity of any of your proteins. Because they often do not know which specific SNPs influence the gene's protein's activity, researchers will often use a SNP that lies close to a gene's coding sequence, and hope that the allele the person has for that SNP can also tell them which alleles that person has for polymorphisms that lie close by.

When two sequences lie very close to each other, it is often true that an individual who has one specific allele of the first sequence will also have a particular allele of the second sequence. In these cases, you can test one SNP as a means of telling what the sequence of the other SNP is, because knowing the person's status for the first SNP tells you what his/her status is for the second SNP. When knowing the person's status for one sequence gives you information about his/her status for a second sequence, the two sequences are said to be **genetically linked**.

If two SNPs are 100% linked, then you can test one SNP as a means of telling what the sequence of the other SNP is. Unfortunately, however, even the most tightly linked SNPs are usually still not in perfect 100% linkage. This means that, while your test will provide accurate information about the critical SNP for most of the people who have the test performed, there will always be some fraction of people for whom the result of the test is going to be deceiving. Further, without actually testing both SNPs, it is impossible for the analyst to determine in any given case whether or not the SNP that was tested is providing accurate information about the SNP whose status it is supposed to reflect. The analyst therefore has no way of knowing which tests are giving accurate information and which are not.

Different Studies Have Disagreed With Respect To The Significance Of Some Alleles

Critics have rightly pointed out that there is a lot of disagreement between different studies in the research literature with respect to just how significantly some risk-increasing alleles increase your risk for the associated disease. One reason why there is a significant amount of disagreement in the published literature at this time is the fact that many of the early research studies focused on one or a few genes, and included a relatively small number of subjects. Many of the research studies that have identified risk-increasing gene alleles are **association studies**. Association studies identify risk-increasing gene alleles for specific diseases by comparing the frequency of specific gene alleles in healthy people versus people who have that specific disease. Many of the early association studies only looked at a single polymorphism, or a few polymorphisms in one gene. If you only study one gene, but your susceptibility to the disease is influenced by the interaction between that gene's protein and other proteins, as well as nongenetic factors, you may have a lot of healthy subjects who possess the risk-increasing allele of the gene you are studying, but do not have the disease, because they do not have the other critical genetic or nongenetic factors. You may fail to identify that risk-increasing allele as a risk-increasing allele, because the number of healthy subjects that have that allele is so high, it doesn't appear to be a risk-increasing allele.

The other big reason for much of the discrepancy in the published literature involves the sizes of the subject pools that have been used in these studies. Because there are so many different genetic and nongenetic factors that influence your susceptibility to a disease, any single genetic factor will usually only influence your level of susceptibility to that disease to a small degree. This means that you need to use a lot of subjects— sometimes thousands—in order to detect the genetic factors that make a small contribution to your level of susceptibility. There are many cases in which one study has identified a risk-increasing allele, but another study has been unable to confirm the association. In many cases, the study that did not identify the allele in question as a risk-increasing allele may have been too small to detect the effect of the risk-increasing allele.

One final methodological detail that has no doubt caused some of the discrepancies in the literature is the fact that different studies have included subjects from different ethnic groups. It is well known that the frequencies of many gene alleles vary between different ethnic groups. A study that includes subjects from an ethnic group in which a risk-increasing allele is present at high frequency may easily identify that allele as a risk-increasing allele, but a study that focuses on an ethnic group in which that allele is rare may fail to confirm the original study's conclusion, simply because the risk-increasing allele was not present in enough people for the statistical analysis to detect an association between that allele and the disease in question. Researchers have taken note of these problems with the earlier research studies, and the more recent studies have been designed to avoid these pitfalls.

The Base Sequence Of A Gene Does Not Tell You About The Gene's Level Of Activity Or Its Interactions With Other Proteins

Recall that the two issues that determine exactly what level of activity you have in any given protein are whether the amino acid sequence of the protein allows it to perform its function at a reasonable level of activity, and how much of that protein the gene is making. As we discussed in Chapter 2, the former depends primarily on the sequence of bases in the gene's coding region, while the latter depends primarily on the sequence of bases that are found in the gene's promoter region and other regulatory sequences.

One of the limitations all genetic tests, including whole-genome sequencing, have is that knowing the sequence of bases in a gene does not tell you everything you need to know about the level of activity in that gene's protein. Knowing the base sequence of a gene's coding region tells you which amino acids are being put into the protein, but it doesn't assure you that the gene is interacting properly with the other proteins that regulate the rate at which the gene is making its protein. When analysts find that the sequence of a gene's promoter region varies from that of the human DNA reference sequence, it is often impossible to confirm that this sequence variant affects production of the protein unless someone specifically tests the possibility in a laboratory.

The level of activity in a typical gene goes up and down in response to your body's changing needs and the changes in your external and internal environment. We are all aware that we have cycles, among them the day-night cycle, the hungry-full cycle and the menstrual cycle. As you go through these cycles, the activity of many of your genes goes up and down. In addition, we all know that our body's needs change as we get older. The activity of many of our genes changes as we age, too. This introduces another complication for those who are interpreting the results of genetic tests: that the significance of some genetic factors may change as you get older.

There is another very important process whereby the level of activity in many genes is regulated: a gene's activity is controlled in part by chemical modifications that get made in the DNA. These chemical modifications are referred to as **epigenetic factors** (see Chapter 7), because they influence the activity of a gene, but do not directly affect the gene's base sequence. One of the epigenetic factors that control the activity of a number of genes involves the adding of chemical groups called methyl groups (chemical formula CH_3) to the C bases that are located in the genes' promoter regions. There have already been inexpensive, reliable assays developed that can measure the degree of methylation in a gene's regulatory sequences. In fact, current research suggests that there may be some cases of colorectal cancer in which measuring the methylation status of the DNA in the tumor tissue can help your doctor decide which treatment may be safest and most effective for you; this is currently being investigated. As we learn more about the way epigenetic factors influence the activity of our genes and proteins, more of the new tests will include assessments of epigenetic factors such as methylation of DNA.

Because almost all proteins work with other proteins to operate the various metabolic pathways your body depends on, the way these proteins interact with each other is often a very important factor influencing the level of activity you have in the protein.

In addition, other types of molecules influence the activity of many of your genes. Future tests will not only determine the individual's status for gene variants, but will also measure the levels of a number of proteins, minerals and electrolytes such as calcium and sodium, and other important molecules, to get the most accurate assessment of how well the relevant biological pathways are working in your body.

Sequencing May Be The Only Way To Capture The Variability In The Human DNA Sequence

As discussed above, testing one SNP that does not influence the activity of a protein itself, but is genetically linked to one that does, can provide important information about someone's risk for a disease. Unfortunately, however, many researchers have made an assumption about the way to interpret the results they obtained using these SNPs that may not be correct, at least in many cases.

Researchers have assumed that, when an association study finds an association between an allele of a linked SNP and a disease, a single polymorphism that lies close to the tested SNP is the critical polymorphism that is influencing the level of activity of that gene's protein. Researchers have assumed that every person in the study who had the risk-increasing SNP allele and the disease (*i.e.* everyone who provided evidence for an association between the SNP allele and the disease) also had the same allele of the critical polymorphism that lies close by the SNP that was tested. In other words, researchers always understood that the linked SNP that was tested was not the critical polymorphism, but they usually assumed that there was one single polymorphism in the region surrounding the linked SNP that was responsible for the association they saw in all the people who had the disease plus the "risk-increasing" allele of the SNP that was tested.

Some researchers have suggested recently, however, that this interpretation might be flawed. They suggest that, instead of there being one single polymorphism in the region around the tested SNP that accounts for all the people who had the disease plus the "risk-increasing" allele of the tested SNP, there are a number of polymorphisms in the region surrounding the SNP, each of which accounts for a few of the people who had the disease plus the "risk-increasing" allele of the tested SNP.

This has important implications when it comes to calculating a person's risk for a disease based on the result of a SNP test. If there actually is a single polymorphism in the identified region that is responsible for everyone's association, then you can give people an accurate estimate of the penetrance of that risk-increasing allele, and give them a reasonably accurate estimate of how strongly possessing that risk-increasing allele increases their probability of developing that disease. If, however, there are a number of different risk-increasing alleles in that region, each of them may have a different level of penetrance. This will make it impossible to provide an accurate estimate regarding how strongly possessing the "risk-increasing" allele of the linked SNP influences the person's risk of developing the disease.

The biggest implication of this is that sequencing may end up being the only way to truly determine which alleles of the critical polymorphisms each individual possesses. Whether you focus on a single gene or sequence the person's entire genome, these findings suggest that the only way to identify each individual's critical genetic factors is to sequence the DNA, and look at the sequence base-by-base. Fortunately, the declining cost of whole-genome sequencing will make this possible in the near future. Not only will sequencing be used routinely in all fields of medicine, it will also be used by more and more researchers, providing huge amounts of data for researchers to work with, causing the already accelerating pace of research in personalised medicine to increase even further.

Whole-Family Sequencing Can Identify Elusive Disease-Causing Mutations

As whole-genome sequencing gets less expensive, the ability to sequence the entire DNA from several members of the same family will help analysts identify which genetic variations contribute to the diseases seen in family members, and which do not. When you know the entire sequence of the DNA from both the parents and their children, you can see exactly which children inherited which gene alleles from the two parents, making it easier to see when a risk-increasing allele or single-gene mutation is reliably associated with a disease.

For example, one family in Utah was reported recently (Salt Lake Tribune, April 22, 2010), in which both children had two rare genetic diseases, Miller syndrome and Primary Ciliary Dyskinesia (PCD). Until this family's DNA was analysed, there were a number of genes that were suspected to be involved in both these diseases. The entire genome was sequenced for both parents and both children, and the results allowed researchers to determine that several of the genes that had been suspected of being involved in these diseases were not actually involved. In fact, if the researchers had merely sequenced the DNA of the two affected children, they would have had 34 gene variants that were potentially the cause of the children's diseases. By sequencing the parents' DNA, however, researchers could track the inheritance of each gene's sequence from parents to children, and this allowed the researchers to narrow down the list of potential genes to only four. One of the four genes was already suspected to be involved in PCD, and this study confirmed that suspicion. After further research, one of the other of the four genes is now believed to be the gene that is primarily responsible for Miller syndrome.

Evan's Story--Whole-Genome SNP Screening In A Man With Type 1 Diabetes And A Family History Of Coronary Heart Disease

Evan was five years old when he was admitted to the emergency department with newly diagnosed type 1 diabetes mellitus (DM1). His blood glucose level was very high and after treatment, he recounts having several weeks of increased thirst, increased urination and weight loss. Because he has DM1, Evan must perform regular fingerprick blood glucose tests on himself, have his hemoglobin A1C monitored, give himself regular insulin injections and get regular medical examinations to check for the many effects diabetes can have on other aspects of your health. Evan is now forty-seven years old, and although he keeps himself in good physical shape, exercises routinely and watches his diet and environmental exposures, he has developed hypertension (high blood pressure), and is worried and anxious about his risk for heart disease and other medical conditions. He also has a significant family history of heart disease in his father and paternal grandfather (his father's father), each of whom had a heart attack in their mid-50s and died soon after. Evan is African-American. Figure 6.3 illustrates Evan's pedigree.

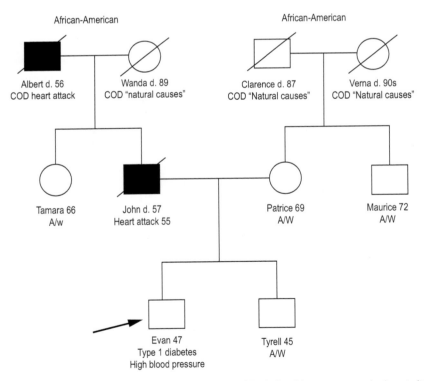

Figure 6.3 Evan's pedigree. A/W = alive and well; COD = cause of death. People's ages or ages at death are indicated.

The Genome-Wide SNP Analysis Provides A Lot Of Information

Evan learns about a company that provides genome-wide SNP analyses through the Internet that are capable of providing information about someone's risk for common diseases such as heart disease, and decides he wants to learn more. He contacts the company, submits a saliva sample and payment, and approximately four weeks later receives an email that his test results are ready for viewing. He goes to the company's website and enters his private account information.

Evan finds that he has quite a number of SNP-associated trait reports to read through, which at first glance is quite overwhelming. For each SNP, the associated results report indicates whether he has one, two or no risk-increasing alleles for that SNP. For example, one SNP tells him that he is a "fast caffeine metaboliser" because he has two copies of the "A" allele of the relevant SNP. This means that drinking relatively large volumes of coffee shouldn't increase his risk for a heart attack, as it can for people who possess the other allele of that SNP. Evan is also pleasantly surprised to learn that he has a lower-than-average risk for asthma, celiac disease, dyslexia and lupus, but the report also states that he has a higher-than-average risk for adult-related macular degeneration (degeneration of the retina in the eye) and psoriasis. Although Evan finds all this information very interesting, he is uncertain what implications these test results have for his prior history of diabetes and high blood pressure, and his future risk for heart disease.

Evan also has one copy of a risk-increasing SNP allele that has been reported to increase your risk for heart disease. This SNP lies in a region of chromosome 9 called 9p21, and it is believed that there are several gene polymorphisms in the 9p21 region that influence your risk for heart disease. While the report clearly states that Evan possesses a SNP allele that increases his risk for heart disease, Evan is uncertain about what to do with this information. He is uncertain what his overall risk for heart disease is, and whether he should change any of his dietary, environmental or lifestyle habits to reduce his exposure to the critical nongenetic factors. He is further confused by the fact that the report states that his risk for DM1 is "typical," when he already has this condition.

Evan's situation is similar to that of other people who have decided to have genetic testing using these direct-to-consumer testing kits. In most cases, the presence of an atypical-risk allele raises more questions than it answers. These tests can tell you that you have a greater-than-average genetic risk for a condition, but they don't tell you what your overall risk is for that disease, because they often don't consider other genetic factors, family history or the critical nongenetic factors. In addition, knowing which gene alleles you possess often doesn't tell you whether you should act on this information by changing your diet, environment or lifestyle, or undergoing early and frequent screening and detection procedures. Without appropriate guidance from a genetic counselor, many people might make decisions about follow up and management based on an incomplete risk picture.

Meeting With The Doctor And Genetic Counselor

Evan decides to bring his entire SNP risk report to his family doctor when he goes for his annual physical examination later that month. His doctor already knows about Evan's family history of heart disease, because Evan provided the doctor access to his family history information during his physical exam last year, after using the Surgeon General's Family History Tool (discussed in Chapter 4). In fact, the doctor has already informed Evan that his prior history of diabetes carries a relative risk of 1.7 for coronary heart disease. This means that Evan is 70% more likely (or 1.7 times as likely) to develop coronary heart disease than someone who is not diabetic. In addition, the doctor has been monitoring Evan's blood lipid (cholesterol and other fats) levels, blood sugar level and body mass index (BMI) regularly, and they have all been normal. The doctor also notes that, because Evan's blood pressure medication is keeping his high blood pressure under control, this additional risk-increasing factor is well controlled.

Evan's doctor has taken some prudent steps to help Evan reduce his risk for heart disease. Because of some conflicting claims in the medical literature, however, the doctor is uncertain exactly how strongly the risk-increasing allele in 9p21 influences Evan's risk for heart disease. The doctor is also not sure whether Evan's family history adds significantly to Evan's risk or not. The doctor decides to refer Evan to a cardiology clinic for a second opinion. Evan's doctor is also uncertain about the value of the other genetic tests in the whole-genome SNP screen, so he feels more comfortable when he learns that the cardiology clinic also has the services of a genetic counselor available.

The genetic counselor and cardiologist meet with Evan during his initial visit. They go through his medical and family history, and the SNP screen report. The genetic counselor explains that even though the commercial testing companies warn that the results of their test should not be used for medical purposes, for some traits and individuals such as Evan, these reports do contain information that can be used to guide their medical decisions.

The first concern is the fact that Evan has a risk-increasing allele in the chromosome 9p21 region. There is a small body of literature that suggests that the risk-increasing allele Evan possesses increases his risk for heart disease by about 15-20%. The cardiologist and genetic counselor know of another recent study, however, that suggested that knowing Evan possess the risk-increasing 9p21 allele does not improve their ability to predict his heart disease risk compared to using the online Framingham risk score tool (discussed in Chapter 4).

The small effect that many of these genetic factors have on your risk for a specific disease makes it hard to interpret the significance of many of these tests. Even if the studies that suggest a 15-20% increase in risk are accurate, if your family history and nongenetic factors put you at a relatively low risk, possessing a risk-increasing gene allele that increases your risk by 15-20% will probably not cause your doctor to recommend that you undertake any special dietary, environmental, or lifestyle changes, or that you undergo any particularly aggressive screening and detection procedures. A 15-20% increase in risk will make a bigger difference, however, for people whose family history and nongenetic factors endow them with a moderate-to-high risk.

Given his significant family history of heart disease, his prior history of diabetes and high blood pressure, and the fact that Evan is over age 40 and a male, he would be considered a high–risk patient, even if he did not possess the risk-increasing 9p21 allele. The cardiologist orders a baseline electrocardiogram (EKG) and additional blood studies, including C-reactive protein and lipid levels, during this initial visit, all of which come back in the normal range.

Designing A Personalised Health Care Plan For Evan

The cardiologist and counselor design a plan to continue to follow Evan every year in the cardiology clinic for follow up EKG and to monitor other heart disease risk factors. Because a review of medical records on Evan's father and grandfather only noted that they had had heart attacks (myocardial infarctions), more specific genetic testing for known single gene diseases that include heart disease among their symptoms is not indicated at the present time. Evan was advised that each of his family members may also be at higher risk for diabetes, high blood pressure and heart disease, and should be monitored for these conditions through their healthcare team. Like Evan, they should avoid the nongenetic factors that increase risk for heart disease, such as smoking and a high-fat diet.

The next concern is the apparent contradiction between the fact that Evan has DM1 and the report's conclusion that Evan has a typical level of risk for DM1. The genetic counselor explains that these genetic tests only give information about some of the genetic factors that are contributing to any given disease. In fact, there are many more genes that influence your risk for DM1 than the one that is reflected in the SNP test, so having a normal result for just one or a few gene polymorphisms can be quite misleading. In addition, the counselor emphasises that nongenetic factors can make a strong contribution to the risk for diabetes, so any gene test available at this time, no matter how complete, only captures a portion of the person's risk factors. Because of this, there are a number of reasons why someone could have typical-risk alleles for the genes that are included in the whole-genome SNP screen, but have other risk-increasing genetic and nongenetic factors that resulted in him/her having DM1.

The other finding that the genetic counselor discusses with Evan is the fact that Evan has a risk-increasing allele for age-related macular degeneration (AMD). This is a disease that causes deterioration of the macula (the central portion of the retina of the eye). Genetic influences account for ~70% of the risk factors for AMD. Individuals with a single relative with AMD have a 2-3 fold increase in risk, while those with two or more relatives are nearly four times as likely to develop AMD as the typical person is. The risk is even higher if the affected family members were diagnosed before the age of 65. The risk-increasing allele that Evan possesses has been seen in almost half of all people with AMD, making it a very common risk factor. If a person is heterozygous (has one copy) for the variant, as Evan is, his/her relative risk is 2.7; the relative risk is 7.0 in people who have two copies of this risk-increasing allele.

Fortunately for Evan, there are a number of important nongenetic factors that he can control his exposure to and reduce his risk of developing AMD. For example, Evan has never smoked, which is one well-known risk-increasing nongenetic factor. In addition, the fact that Evan has kept his weight under control avoids another risk-increasing genetic factor, obesity. There are also a number of preventive measures Evan can take to help reduce his risk for AMD. Wearing sunglasses that protect the eyes by blocking the sun's ultraviolet (UV) rays reduces the risk for AMD. He can also influence his risk for AMD through dietary measures. This includes eating a balanced diet that includes leafy green vegetables, as well as supplementing his diet with an eye-specific antioxidant vitamin supplement containing the established dosages of vitamins A, C and E, as well as zinc, selenium and copper. In addition, the supplemental antioxidants lutein and zeaxanthin, which are being investigated as possible risk-reducing factors, are often contained in these supplements. Lutein and zeaxanthin are the pigments contained in green leafy vegetables such as spinach, kale and collard greens. Taking a daily low-dose aspirin may also have a preventive effect, possibly because of aspirin's anti-inflammatory activity. This may provide Evan a double benefit, because the aspirin may also help reduce Evan's risk for heart attack and stroke. Finally, it was also recommended that Evan be referred to an ophthalmologist for routine eye exams and follow up.

IT IS IMPORTANT FOR YOU TO BE AN INFORMED CONSUMER

As you can see, there are a lot of potential benefits to be gained from genetic testing, but there are also some serious issues that may arise if you choose to have genetic testing.

Genetic counselors can help you with many aspects of this process, from understanding exactly what the genetic tests look at to recommending a plan for maintaining your health as effectively as possible after you receive the results of the testing. In many cases, knowing which diseases you have a higher than average genetic risk for may help you adjust your diet, environment and lifestyle to reduce your exposure to the critical nongenetic factors. Even if your genetic risk is so high that there may be little you can do to prevent the disease from developing, you may still be able to undergo a more personalised schedule of screening and detection procedures, which may enable your doctor to detect the disease early enough to treat it successfully.

As the field of personalised medicine matures, the tests that emerge will provide ever more useful information, and will be increasingly able to help your doctor make more accurate diagnoses, predict your risk for specific diseases more accurately and choose the treatment that will be safest and most effective for you. In the future, as more genetic testing companies advertise their services directly to consumers, it will become increasingly important for you to understand the potential benefits and limitations of genetic testing, so you can determine whether the benefits of the new tests justify the costs and potential impact of genetic testing.

Chapter Summary

- Personalised medicine enables you--even expects you--to take a more active role in maintaining your own health, as well as making decisions regarding your health care.

- There are many issues to consider before you decide to have genetic testing performed. They include cost, privacy of the information, potential benefit, potential psychological and emotional impact and the significance of the information for your family members.

- There are several reasons why it can be difficult to interpret the results of a genetic test. There are a great many sequence variations in the typical person's DNA that do not impact the individual's health. In addition, it can be difficult to determine exactly what effect a sequence variation can have on the level of activity of that gene or that gene's protein.

- While some genetic testing companies provide educational material on their website, it is often beneficial to speak with or meet with a genetic counselor to get help interpreting the significance of the results of a genetic test.

- Because the human DNA sequence is so highly variable, whole-genome sequencing may be the only way to identify all the risk-increasing and risk-decreasing gene alleles someone has.

- Whole-family sequencing, in which whole-genome sequencing is performed on the parents and all children from a family, can be very helpful in identifying gene sequence variants that are responsible for disease.

CHAPTER 7

NUTRIGENOMICS AND EPIGENETICS: THE EFFECTS OUR DIET, ENVIRONMENT AND LIFESTYLE HAVE ON OUR GENES AND PROTEINS

WHAT YOU EAT AFFECTS THE LEVEL OF ACTIVITY IN SOME OF YOUR GENES AND PROTEINS

Most people would agree that good nutrition helps keep us healthy. In fact, Hippocrates himself[1] proposed that good nutrition could serve as a substitute for medicine for maintaining one's health. As the focus of personalised medicine has expanded from genetics to genomics in the last decade, it has become more apparent that the foods we eat can affect the level of activity in our genes and our proteins in ways that influence our risks of developing specific diseases.

For example, one reason why your diet should contain a high level of antioxidants is that your metabolism and other factors, such as smoking, cause your body to produce harmful chemicals called superoxide radicals. These chemicals damage tissues, and are thought to contribute to a number of multifactorial diseases. Your body has several proteins that break down these superoxide radicals and prevent them from damaging your tissues, including one protein called MnSOD. One reason why selenium is included in many multivitamins is that selenium helps the gene that makes MnSOD work at a higher level of activity. There are several known places in the *MnSOD* gene where the sequence is known to be variable. People with a low-activity allele of the *MnSOD* gene may need to be especially careful to consume an appropriate amount of selenium, to avoid a further increase in their risk of developing certain diseases.

Several other recent studies have shown how dietary advice can be tailored to the individual's genetic status. For example, one study has suggested that people with low-activity alleles of the *GSTM1* gene, whose protein also detoxifies superoxide radicals, must be careful to consume high levels of antioxidants to help reduce their risk of developing several types of cancer. In addition, people who have a high-activity version of the *ACE* gene, whose protein helps increase your blood pressure, may benefit

---

[1] Hippocrates was an ancient Greek physician; he is generally regarded as the founder of the field of medicine.

from consuming certain proteins (*e.g.* pork or soybean extracts), because your body metabolises these proteins into compounds that can reduce the activity of the *ACE* gene.

The field of **nutrigenomics** is among the newest branches of personalised medicine, and at the present time there are very few tests that have been developed that can be used to design personalised nutrition plans. The field is growing quickly, however, and will ultimately be the branch of personalised medicine that has the greatest potential to help the greatest number of people. As genomic researchers learn more about the effects our diet, environment and lifestyle have on our genes and proteins, it is becoming increasingly obvious that these choices have consequences, not only for our health, but in some cases, for the health of our children (discussed below).

We Have Recently Become Aware Of The Importance Of Epigenetic Factors

Genetic researchers have historically been concerned with the way changes in the sequence of bases in a gene's coding sequence influence the activity level of that gene's protein. As we discussed in Chapter 2, when two people have different sequences (alleles) in a gene's coding region, one person may make a version of the protein that has a higher level of activity than the other person's has. As an analogy, imagine two rooms, each of which is lit by a light bulb. Imagine that the two light bulbs have different wattage ratings. When you throw the light switches on in the two rooms, the same amount of electricity is fed into the two light bulbs. The room with the higher-watt bulb will be brighter, however, because the two versions of the light bulbs have different levels of brightness. Similarly, if two people make the same amount of a protein, but one person's version of the protein has greater activity than the other's, that person will have a higher level of activity of that protein in his/her body than the other person will.

There is another way in which differences in two people's gene sequences can influence the level of activity in their proteins. If the level of activity in one person's gene is higher than the level of activity in the other person's gene, that person will make more of that protein, and therefore will have more of that protein's activity in his/her body. For an analogy, imagine two rooms, each of which is lit by a light bulb that has a dimmer switch. Each of the two light bulbs has the same wattage rating, but if the dimmer switch is set to a higher point in one room than the other, that room will have more light in it. Figure 7.1 summarises the two different ways in which the level of activity in a gene's protein can be regulated. The top portion of the figure illustrates the way two different alleles of the gene can cause different people to make versions of the protein that have different amino acid sequences, and therefore different levels of activity. The bottom portion of the figure illustrates how two people can make the same version of the protein, but one person's gene can be working at a higher level of activity than the other person's gene is working, giving that person more of the protein.

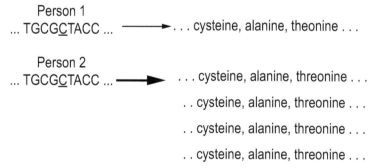

The level of activity you have in a protein at any given time is determined by:

The coding sequence of the gene

Person 1
... TGCG<u>C</u>TACC ... ⟶ ... cysteine, alanine, theonine ...

Person 2
... TGCG<u>A</u>TACC ... ⟶ ... cysteine, histidine, threonine ...

Alanine (small, no electrical charge) version has typical activity

Histidine (large, positive charge) version has lower level of activity

The level of activity of the gene

Person 1
... TGCG<u>C</u>TACC ... ⟶ ... cysteine, alanine, theonine ...

Person 2
... TGCG<u>C</u>TACC ... ⟶ ... cysteine, alanine, threonine ...

.. cysteine, alanine, threonine ...

.. cysteine, alanine, threonine ...

.. cysteine, alanine, threonine ...

Figure 7.1. The level of activity in any given protein is regulated by both the coding sequence and the rate of activity in the corresponding gene.

One way in which the level of activity in a gene is regulated involves **epigenetic factors**. The term "epigenetics" refers to factors that influence the level of activity at which the gene is working without changing the sequence of bases in the gene. Genomic researchers are still discovering many of the epigenetic factors that regulate the activity of our genes, but the best known epigenetic factor involves a chemical reaction that puts a methyl group (chemical formula = CH_3) onto some of the C bases in the gene's promoter region. You will recall from Chapter 2 that the promoter region is the stretch of DNA where specialised proteins bind to control the rate at which the gene is making its protein. In the light bulb analogy above, the promoter region is the dimmer switch, and the proteins that bind to the promoter region of the gene are the hand that sets the dimmer switch to the desired level of power. Putting an excessive number of methyl groups on the C bases in a gene's promoter region interferes with the ability of these proteins to bind to the gene's promoter region. This will reduce the level of activity in the gene, perhaps to the point where the gene is turned off completely.

While both copies of most of your genes are active, you have a number of genes for which you are only supposed to have one active copy (referred to as **imprinted** genes). Many of these genes have a lot of C bases in their promoter region, and in many of these genes, the inactive copy of the gene is turned off by having methyl groups placed on the C bases in its promoter region. Figure 7.2 illustrates how one copy of a gene can be silenced by the methylation of its promoter region's C bases.

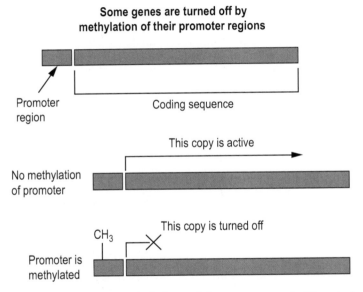

Figure 7.2. For some genes, one copy is turned off when methyl groups are put on the C bases in the gene's promoter region.

Your body's normal pattern of gene regulation includes a certain amount of methylation-induced gene silencing. Too much or too little methylation, however, can result in certain genes working at abnormally high or low rates of activity. Abnormal methylation is thought to be one of the key changes that happen as certain cancers develop. You have proteins that kill cells that have suffered DNA damage, and therefore have an increased risk of becoming cancerous. Because they prevent the growth of cancerous tumors, these proteins, and the genes that produce them, are referred to as **tumor suppressor** proteins and genes. If you increase the level of methylation in these tumor suppressor genes, you can reduce their level of activity, thereby increasing the person's risk for a number of different types of cancer.

Several Types Of Nutrients Influence The Activity Of Your Genes Through Epigenetic Mechanisms

There are a number of chemical processes that occur in your body that depend on a supply of methyl groups to be transferred from one chemical to another. Several essential nutrients help maintain your body's supply of methyl groups. These include vitamin B9 (also known as folate or folic acid), vitamin B12 (cyanocobalamin), vitamin B2 (riboflavin), vitamin B6 (pyridoxal phosphate), the amino acid methionine and the mineral zinc. In addition, some foods contain nutrients that, while not essential, help insure that your body has an adequate supply of methyl groups.

Folate is the most extensively studied of these nutrients. A diet that is high in folate provides many health benefits, and several of these have been linked to changes in epigenetic modification and gene activity. The best known of these is the fact that a deficiency of folate during the period shortly before and shortly after conception increases the child's risk of being born with a neural tube defect such as spina bifida (in which the spine does not close properly, possibly leaving the spinal cord exposed).

Folate also appears to protect people from colorectal cancer, and perhaps other cancers as well. Several studies that measured folate consumption and colon cancer rates in large numbers of people have suggested that a diet that is high in folate can reduce your risk of developing colorectal cancer. In animal models, it has been shown that a high-folate diet can change the level of methylation of certain cancer-related genes. These animal model studies have established a direct link between the level of folate in the diet, the level of activity in specific genes and the risk for colorectal cancer.

Your level of folate consumption may interact with your genetic status, and your level of riboflavin consumption, to influence the level of methylation in your DNA. The folate you eat gets processed chemically by several of your body's proteins, including one that is referred to as MTHFR. Riboflavin helps the MTHFR protein do its work, so your level of riboflavin intake may directly influence the activity of MTHFR. In addition, the *MTHFR* gene has several variants in it that may influence the level of activity in the MTHFR protein.

The most extensively studied variant in the *MTHFR* gene is a C/T SNP in the coding sequence. While most people have a C base at that position, some people have a T base. The C allele makes a version of the protein that has the amino acid alanine as the 222nd amino acid, while the T allele makes a version of the protein that has valine as its 222nd amino acid. Having valine in that position reduces the activity of the protein; MTHFR activity is reduced by 70% in people who have two T alleles for the *MTHFR* gene. Possessing one or more T alleles of the MTHFR gene increases your risk of being born with a neural tube defect (*e.g.* spina bifida) or developing cardiovascular (heart) disease as you age. Both these effects can be counteracted by supplementing the diet with folate.

The way your body processes folate is influenced by a complex interaction between your *MTHFR* genotype, your riboflavin status, and perhaps even your alcohol consumption as well. One study has suggested that if you give people a low-dose folate supplement, adding some riboflavin along with the folate can increase the level of folate you see in those people's blood. People who have two C alleles for the *MTHFR* gene will not get this benefit from the riboflavin, however; only people with the CT or TT genotype will. The situation is further complicated by the fact that several studies have suggested that a high level of alcohol intake can reduce the beneficial effects of a high-folate diet.

There is a growing list of "functional foods" that are thought to reduce people's risks for several different diseases. As genomic researchers expand their studies to include the effects of foods on our genes, they are discovering that many of these functional foods either increase or decrease the activity of specific genes. There have been many studies done using animal models, and a growing body of studies that looked at people. Together, these studies have established several direct links between consumption of a food, changes in the epigenetic modifications of specific genes, changes in the activity levels of these genes, and changes in the individual's risk of developing a specific disease.

For example, nutritional studies suggest that eating soy products (*e.g.* tofu, tempeh, natto, miso) reduces a man's risk for prostate cancer, and may also reduce a premenopausal woman's risk for breast cancer. It is thought that soy contains a group of chemicals called isoflavones that are capable of having several different effects on your metabolism. A number of research studies have shown that a high-isoflavone diet can increase and decrease the activity of certain genes in ways that are expected to reduce a person's risk for prostate cancer. Some have reported that these changes in activity are due to changes in the epigenetic modifications of these genes.

One of the ways in which isoflavones are thought to affect your metabolism involves their ability to bind to the same proteins that female hormones such as estrogen and estradiol bind to. Consistent with this, several studies have reported that variations in genes whose proteins carry these hormones through the bloodstream, or act as the receptor proteins through which these hormones exert their effects on your body, influence the degree to which a high-soy diet will reduce someone's risk of developing cancer.

The fact that isoflavones may increase the activity of estrogen-related systems illustrates the fact that, like prescription drugs, functional foods have the potential for dangerous side effects in certain genetically predisposed people as well. It has recently been discovered that estradiol or other forms of estrogen can increase the risk for a second cancer in some women who have had breast cancer. There is clearly a need for further research in this area, but it is possible that estrogen-sensitive women may be well advised to avoid soy products, while other women may find that eating soy reduces their risk for breast cancer.

THE TYPES OF BACTERIA THAT LIVE IN YOUR DIGESTIVE SYSTEM CAN INFLUENCE THE EFFECTS CERTAIN NUTRIENTS HAVE ON YOUR HEALTH

Isoflavones also illustrate another principle that will no doubt become increasingly important in the field of nutrigenomics. Like many other nutrients, isoflavones are metabolised by the bacteria that live in your digestive system (called your **gut flora**). The typical person's digestive system contains approximately one quadrillion (1,000,000,000,000,000) individual bacteria. There are between 500-1,000 different strains of bacteria that are capable of living in the human digestive system, although 30-40 strains make up the majority of our gut flora. These bacteria are essential to our health. They provide us with the essential vitamins vitamin K and biotin, they make hormones that help regulate fat metabolism, and they help our immune system function, among other things.

In addition to your actual diet and your status for genes whose proteins metabolise your food, the specific strains of bacteria that live in your gut provide another important source of variability in different people's nutritional status. Different people will often have different combinations of strains of bacteria in their systems. This means that different people's gut flora will take the same food and make different chemical byproducts out of it. For example, some people's gut flora produce more of the byproduct equol after they eat soy than other people's do. A high-soy diet has been shown to produce more favorable shifts in hormone levels in high equol producers than in other people. Consequently, high equol producers may reap more health benefits, *e.g.* a greater reduction in their risk for prostate or breast cancer, than other people do from a high-soy diet.

The specific bacteria in your gut flora may also influence your risk for Crohn's disease (CD) and inflammatory bowel disease (IBD). One factor that is thought to influence your risk for these diseases is the way your immune system reacts to the bacteria in your digestive system. Your immune system will respond to different bacteria differently, so it is quite possible that certain gut bacteria can increase a person's risk of developing CD or IBD to a greater degree than other bacteria will. Sequence variants in several genes whose proteins work as part of your immune system have been shown to influence your risk for CD and IBD as well. One of these risk-increasing alleles has a frequency of 25-35% in Europeans, but has a near-zero frequency in Asians and Africans. This may partially explain why the incidence of CD and IBD is considerably higher in people of European descent than it is in Asians or Africans.

GENETICS AND GENOMICS ARE ACTIVE TOPICS IN OBESITY RESEARCH

It is well known that people from certain ethnic groups have a greater probability of becoming obese than others. Some of these groups have evolved in conditions where the availability of key nutrients differed greatly between the harvest season and the leaner seasons. It is thought that evolution favored people whose bodies could store fat more efficiently during the plentiful seasons, thereby providing them a larger energy store for the lean seasons. During the early days of that group's evolution, individuals with efficient fat-storing genes survived longer, were generally healthier, and produced more children than the other members of their group. Consequently, the present-day members of that ethnic group have gene alleles that maximise the amount of fat the body stores from the food you eat.

Nutritional conditions can change within a year, but changing the frequency of certain gene alleles in a population takes generations. When a people who have evolved in conditions of feast and famine find themselves in a situation in which the food supply is more stable, their genes work to store as much fat as possible from their food all year long, resulting in a high incidence of obesity in that ethnic group.

The earliest studies in this field focused on finding gene variants that influenced a person's risk of developing obesity. Because your level of body fat is controlled by the interaction of several of your hormones, genes whose proteins help your hormones perform their functions were natural candidates for study. Your hormones exert their effects on your body by binding to specific proteins called receptors. Variations in several of the genes that make hormone receptor proteins have been found to influence the level of fat in your body in general, as well as a woman's predisposition to retain weight after pregnancy. Variations in the sequences of genes such as these can have consequences for many aspects of your metabolism. In fact, one of the alleles of a gene called *GNB3* increases your risk, not only of developing obesity, but of developing atherosclerosis, as well as metabolic syndrome, which includes high blood pressure, high blood cholesterol and resistance to insulin.

Your genetics also influences how your body responds to you being overweight. The cells in which we store most of our fat serve several other purposes for metabolism. They release hormones that help regulate your appetite and metabolism, and they also release chemicals that cause inflammation. Obesity is accompanied by low-level inflammation throughout the body, because an obese person's fat-storing cells release excessive amounts of these inflammation-causing chemicals. Inflammation causes damage to several different types of tissues, and is thought to contribute to many multifactorial diseases. Sequence variations in several genes influence how much of these inflammation-causing chemicals get released from your fat-storing cells. People who are obese and possess certain alleles of these genes will experience even more inflammation, and thereby increase their risk for several diseases to an even greater degree, than other obese people will.

A similar finding has been reported regarding the risk of developing type 2 diabetes upon becoming obese. One of the alleles of a gene whose protein regulates your body's sensitivity to insulin has been shown to influence an obese person's risk of developing type 2 diabetes.

Your genetic factors also control your response to certain weight-reducing drugs. For example, variations in the sequences of the *GNB3*, *GNAS* and *GNA11* genes influence your response to the weight-reducing drug sibutramine. People who possess certain alleles of these genes lose more weight than others when given sibutramine. In addition, the specific alleles the person has for the *GNAS* gene influence his/her risk of experiencing significant changes in heart rate in response to the drug. Tests that assess the person's status for these genes can make weight-loss interventions safer and more effective.

As the field of personalised medicine has expanded from genetics to genomics, several recent studies have shown that a high-fat diet alters the activity of certain genes in ways that help explain why a high-fat diet has negative consequences for your health. Much of the danger seems to lie in the fact that, when your body metabolises fats, it creates chemicals called reactive oxygen species (ROS, aka superoxide radicals), which can damage several types of tissues and contribute to many multifactorial diseases.

In a number of studies that used animal models, a high-fat diet reduced the level of activity in several genes whose proteins break down fats to harvest energy from them. Supplementing the diet with the antioxidant lipoic acid counteracted this effect, and restored the level of activity in these genes. Lipoic acid also reduced the level of activity in several genes whose proteins help synthesise cholesterol. In addition to these effects on fat metabolism, lipoic acid also increased the activity of several genes whose proteins detoxify the ROS that are generated when your body metabolises fats.

One goal of nutrigenetic researchers is to be able to give people dietary recommendations that are based on the individual's genetic makeup. One published study has reported that people who had genetic testing performed, then were given personalised advice based on the results, reduced their blood sugar levels to a greater degree, lost more weight and maintained their weight loss for longer than people who had been put on a standard healthy diet. The genetic testing and dietary recommendations were not designed for weight loss; they were designed to provide each individual the best balance of nutrients possible. The people in the study had all failed at previous weight loss efforts, however, and were all significantly overweight. The genetic test looked at variants in 19 genes whose proteins help regulate several different aspects of our metabolism. Table 7-1 illustrates some of the dietary recommendations that were given to people based on the predicted effects their genetic status had on their metabolism.

Table 7-1. Dietary Recommendations Given To People Based On The Results Of Their Genetic Tests*

Effect of gene variants on metabolism	Recommendation
Impaired metabolism of folate, reduced supply of methyl groups	Add folic acid, vitamin B6 and vitamin B12
Reduced ability to detoxify cancer-causing agents, prescription drugs, environmental toxins and reactive oxygen species	Increase cruciform vegetables such as broccoli, cauliflower, Brussels sprouts, kale, cabbage, and bok choy Increase allium vegetables such as onions and garlic
Reduced antioxidant activity	Add antioxidant vitamins such as A, C and E
Increased risk for age-related bone loss	Reduce caffeine, increase dairy foods, add vitamin D and calcium
Increased level of inflammation in the body	Increase omega-3 fats, both dietary sources (oily fish) and supplements

* From Arkadianos *et al.*, Nutrition Journal, 6:29. (2007)

A Pregnant Woman's Nutritional State Can Affect The Activity Of Her Child's Genes

Improper Maternal Nutrition May Increase The Child's Risk For Several Diseases

We all know that if a pregnant woman does not get proper nutrition it may have negative consequences for her child's health. For example, it is well established that maternal undernutrition can decrease the child's birth weight. A low birth weight increases your risk for several diseases, including high blood pressure, heart disease, high cholesterol and type 2 diabetes. In addition, children who were conceived during the severe famine that plagued The Netherlands in the winter of 1944-1945 have now been shown to have an increased risk of developing several diseases, despite having normal birth weights. The diseases for which these people have an increased risk include not only metabolic diseases such as high body mass index, high blood fats and cardiovascular disease, but also psychological diseases such as schizophrenia.

Improper maternal nutrition includes not only situations in which the mother is undernourished, but also situations in which the mother is overnourished, obese, or has a disease of her own metabolism, such as diabetes. Both clinical and animal model studies have shown that the children of an obese mother have an increased risk of being obese and having metabolic diseases (high blood fats, diabetes) themselves. In addition, animal studies have reported that the degree to which the offspring are overweight may increase from generation to generation, but that supplementing the mother's diet with things that insure an adequate supply of methyl groups can stop the cycle of increasing obesity.

If the mother has a metabolic disease, this can result in the child having an improper nutritional environment while in the womb, despite the mother consuming a proper diet. This may cause the child's metabolism to shift as well. This shift in the child's metabolism will change the way the child's body processes nutrients over the entire course of the child's life. This in turn will have consequences for the child's health over the course of his/her lifetime. For example, children whose mothers have high blood sugar have an increased risk of developing several types of metabolic diseases, especially type 2 diabetes.

Research studies using animal models have shed a lot of light on the mechanisms whereby prenatal influences affect one's health later in life. These studies suggest that there are two ways in which the mother's nutritional status can affect the activity of her child's genes (Figure 7.3). First, if improper nutrition or a metabolic disease causes abnormal methylation of the mother's DNA, these epigenetic changes may be inherited directly by her children, and affect the activity of some of their genes.

Alternatively, a number of researchers have suggested that the child's metabolism gets adjusted as if the child's body predicts that the nutritional environment it will be in after it is born is the same as the nutritional environment it is in before it is born. If the mother has a metabolic disorder, this will cause the mother's blood to contain amounts of proteins, fats, sugars and other important nutrients that are different from the amounts that are usually present when someone consumes a balanced diet. While the child is in the womb, it may receive excess amounts of some nutrients from the mother's blood, and/or it may be deprived of other important nutrients. This may change the level of activity of some of the child's genes, to levels that are appropriate for someone who will receive that same balance of nutrients throughout his/her entire life. This includes genes whose proteins metabolise our energy-rich foods (such as fats and carbohydrates), regulate how much fat our body stores, or help our hormones perform their functions, one of which is to regulate our metabolism. If, after the child is born, he/she consumes a more balanced diet, his/her body may not process the food appropriately, because the level of activity in the genes whose proteins metabolise our food have been set to levels that are more appropriate for a different balance of proteins, fats, sugars and other nutrients.

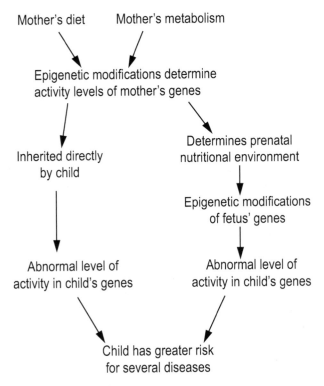

Figure 7.3. Two mechanisms whereby the nutritional environment the child experiences in the womb can affect the child's health later in life.

Recent Research Has Demonstrated The Importance Of Epigenetic Changes

There is mounting evidence that some of the effects of maternal undernutrition, overnutrition or metabolic diseases may be linked to the child having abnormal methylation (or other epigenetic modifications), and therefore an abnormally high or low level of activity, in certain genes. Research using animal models has shown that putting pregnant mothers on a low-protein diet can alter the level of methylation, and the level of activity, in several genes. This includes genes that make some of the proteins that help regulate your blood pressure, the function of your body's hormones, and several aspects of your metabolism, including blood sugar transport, fat storage and fat metabolism. There have been many different types of studies done, using rodents, sheep and even monkeys. Together these studies have provided a direct link between improper nutrition in the mother, altered epigenetic modifications in the offspring's DNA, increased and decreased activity in specific genes in the offspring and the offspring's increased risk for specific metabolic diseases. Further, several of these studies have shown that supplementing the mother's diet with folate or other things that increase her supply of methyl groups, or leptin, a hormone that helps regulate fat metabolism, can prevent or reverse these effects of maternal undernutrition.

In addition to maternal undernutrition, it also appears that maternal overnutrition and obesity may also change the epigenetic modifications, and level of activity, of several genes. Several animal studies, including one study using monkeys, have shown changes in epigenetic factors, and both decreases and increases in the activity level of specific genes, in the offspring of mothers who were kept on high-fat diets. These studies have also shown that this effect can be prevented if you supplement the mother's diet with nutrients that help insure an adequate supply of methyl groups, such as folate.

While we are obviously limited in our ability to perform research using human subjects, several research groups have found ways to study the relationship between maternal nutrition and the child's epigenetic state directly. Situations in which the availability of nutrients is extremely variable from one season to another allow researchers to assess the effects of maternal undernutrition on people's genes. One study that was conducted in rural Gambia reported that children who were conceived during the nutrition-poor season (July-November) have lower birth weights and shorter life spans than children born at other times of the year. In addition, they show higher levels of methylation in specific genes, but not in their DNA in general.

The "Hunger Winter" that plagued The Netherlands in the winter of 1944-1945 also provided researchers the opportunity to study the effects of maternal undernutrition on the child's epigenetics. Researchers have reported both increases and decreases in the methylation of specific genes in people who were conceived before or during the famine. The men who had been conceived during the famine also had an increased frequency of being born with the neural tube defect spina bifida (in which the spine does not close properly). This is particularly interesting from an epigenetic standpoint, because it is well established that a deficiency of folate, specific gene variants, and other things that reduce the supply of methyl groups during the period just before and just after conception increase the child's risk of being born with a neural tube defect.

While most of the attention has been focused on situations of extreme maternal malnutrition or obesity, some researchers have recently shown that the relationship between maternal nutrition, methylation of the child's genes and the child's metabolism also holds for the normally nourished population. This implies that the principles of nutrigenomics may be applicable to all people, not just to those who had to cope with extremely abnormal prenatal environments. One recent series of studies has looked at the methylation of DNA from a series of healthy newborns' umbilical cords. This study reported that children whose mothers had the lowest levels of carbohydrate intake had the highest levels of body fat and the highest levels of methylation in the promoter region of a gene called *RXRA*. The RXRA protein controls the level of activity of several genes whose proteins regulate your fat metabolism and your sensitivity to insulin; changes in *RXRA* activity could easily provide a link between maternal carbohydrate consumption and the child's metabolism.

The interactions between nutrients and genes are highly complicated; it will take some time and research before we understand them well enough to incorporate these principles into routine practice. For example, recent studies suggest that the effects of an improper fetal nutritional environment depend on the sex of the child and the period during which the child was exposed. Both human and animal studies have reported that the severity of the effects differ in male versus female offspring. Most studies report that male offspring are more sensitive to the effects of prenatal malnutrition than female offspring, although there have been a few effects that were observed only in females.

These studies also suggest that there are several time periods during which an individual's epigenetic status can be changed. It is clear that DNA methylation and gene activity are extremely sensitive to the fetus' nutritional environment during the period surrounding the child's conception. This means that it is especially important for women who are planning to get pregnant to begin a proper nutritional regimen before they get pregnant. It is not just the period around conception that is important, however. Research studies also report that exposure to an improper nutritional environment later in the pregnancy can cause epigenetic changes that have negative consequences for the offspring's health.

The prenatal period is not the only period during which epigenetic changes occur. Your DNA undergoes epigenetic changes throughout your entire life span. The changes in epigenetic DNA modifications and gene activity that occur progressively as you go through your later years may in fact be part of the reason why elderly people have increased risks of developing certain diseases. Several studies have shown that the level of methylation in our DNA is generally reduced as we get older. A decrease in methylation has been shown to occur in a number of specific genes. In addition, however, an increase in methylation, and a reduction of activity, has been reported in several tumor suppressor genes and other cancer-related genes. This may explain why elderly people have an increased risk of developing a number of different types of cancer. Other studies have also shown that the methylation of two genes whose proteins are involved in the process by which we harvest energy from fats and carbohydrates is increased in elderly people. This increased methylation reduces the level of activity in both these genes, and the reductions in activity paralleled the decreases in insulin sensitivity that were seen in these people.

WHAT THE FATHER EATS AND DRINKS MAY ALSO INFLUENCE GENE ACTIVITY IN THE CHILD

Most of the focus has been on the mother's diet, environment and lifestyle, but researchers have recently begun studying the effects that a father's diet, environment and lifestyle can have on his children's genes as well. For example, it is already known that having an obese father increases your risk for obesity, and having a father with insulin resistance or diabetes increases your risk for diabetes. One recent study has suggested that, just like maternal obesity, these effects may be mediated through changes in methylation of the children's genes. These researchers reported that feeding male rats a high-fat diet reduced insulin secretion, reduced the number of beta cells in the pancreas (which secrete insulin), and changed the methylation pattern of one of the genes in their daughters' DNA. More research is clearly needed to determine the influence that paternal factors such as diet have on the activity of their children's genes.

Paternal drinking is not thought to disrupt the child's development the way maternal drinking does. Animal studies have established, however, that paternal alcohol consumption can have a number of negative effects on the children's mental and physical development. Several of these studies have demonstrated that paternal alcohol consumption results in a reduced level of methylation in several genes, which can increase the level of activity in these genes.

One recent study using human volunteers confirmed that high alcohol intake resulted in reduced methylation of the genes in men's sperm cells. The genes that were studied belong to a class of genes called imprinted genes. Although you inherit two copies of each imprinted gene, one copy is silenced, often by methylation of the promoter region in that copy of the gene. For the two genes that were studied, the copy that is inherited from the father is heavily methylated and silenced. Reduced methylation can activate these normally silenced copies of these genes. You have a number of imprinted genes for which the copy you inherited from your father is silenced, so this can have a number of negative consequences for the child's development.

At this point there are only a few studies that have tried to determine how fathers' diets, environments and lifestyles can affect the activity of their children's genes. These studies suggest that these paternal factors work in a manner similar to the maternal factors, by altering the epigenetic modification of the father's genes. This can change the level at which the gene is working in the fetus, and disturb the fetus' development in a number of ways. This is clearly an area where more research is needed.

Keeping Your Chromosome Telomeres Long May Help Keep You Healthier As You Age

The ends of your chromosomes are called the **telomeres**. The telomeres have a special structure that keeps your chromosomes from degrading and maintains the appropriate level of activity in many of your genes. As you get older, however, your telomeres get shorter. Several studies have suggested that the shortening of your telomeres is one reason why your risk of developing specific diseases such as cancer, cardiovascular disease, Parkinson disease and Alzheimer disease increases as you get older. The rate at which your telomeres shorten may also influence your life span.

There are several aspects of your metabolism that appear to influence the rate at which your telomeres shorten as you age. Nutrients that increase the supply of methyl groups, reduce inflammation or have antioxidant activity (*e.g.* folate, vitamin B12, the amino acid methionine, vitamins C and E) all slow the rate at which your telomeres shrink.

One of the best-known factors that speeds up the rate of telomere shrinkage is stress. There have been a number of studies that have reported finding shorter telomeres in people who had been subjected to various types of stress. The stresses included being raised in an orphanage, being a victim of domestic violence, having an overbearing work schedule and post-traumatic stress disease after childhood trauma. Interestingly, while it is well known that chronic poverty and other negative economic factors are stressful, in the studies that measured socioeconomic status, it did not appear to affect the length of people's telomeres the way emotional/psychological stressors did.

The fact that your level of stress can influence the shortening of your telomeres represents a point at which all people can help improve the quality of their own health as they age. By reducing your stress level and managing stress properly, you can slow the rate at which your telomeres shorten, and potentially reduce your risk of developing a number of diseases as you age.

There are several companies that offer telomere length tests, but many experts question whether these tests are truly useful. These tests cannot specify the diseases for which you may have an increased risk. They also cannot tell you how long you can expect to live. Even if the test reveals that you have excessively short telomeres, there have not been any drugs developed yet that can increase your telomere length. Some commentators have suggested that it is better to recommend that people save themselves the cost of the test, and just reduce their level of stress and maintain a diet that has plenty of antioxidants and insures a good supply of methyl groups, for this and many other reasons.

THE FIELD OF NUTRIGENOMICS WILL IMPACT PERSONALISED MEDICINE IN A NUMBER OF WAYS

There is a lot of research being conducted in the field of nutrigenomics, and researchers will undoubtedly discover many ways in which our genetics and diet influence each other in the near future. As the field progresses, researchers will also study how a person's ethnic origin, age and other factors interact with diet and genetics. In the not-too-distant future, genetic/genomic tests will be developed that can be used to design diets that reduce people's risks of developing disease such as coronary artery disease, diabetes, high blood pressure, arthritis and asthma. In addition, nutrigenomics and pharmacogenomics will become more integrated in the future. Not only will drug therapies become more personalised, but drug prescriptions will also be accompanied by recommendations about diet that are tailored to the individual's genetic status. Researchers are also studying the effects that exercise has on the activity levels of our genes; recommendations for exercise plans will be integrated with dietary recommendations and drug prescriptions.

CHAPTER SUMMARY

- Early studies focused on the effects our gene variants have on the processing of our foods, but more recently the focus has expanded to include the effects our foods have on the activity of our genes.

- Researchers have recently become aware that the epigenetic modifications that regulate the level of activity in our genes are highly variable between different people, and play an important role in determining our risk for diseases.

- A number of essential nutrients and functional foods help insure an adequate supply of methyl groups; this has been shown to affect the methylation status and level of activity of specific genes.

- Another source of variability in people's nutritional status lies in the fact that different people have different strains of bacteria in their digestive system. The specific bacteria you have in your gut may determine the degree of benefit you will get from certain functional foods, and may influence your risk for inflammatory bowel disease and Crohn's disease as well.

- With the growing concerns over obesity, considerable research is focused on determining both the genetic factors that contribute to obesity and the effects of obesity on the activity of our genes. One study has demonstrated that providing people personalised dietary recommendations based on the results of genetic tests increases the degree to which they reduce their blood sugar and the amount and duration of their weight loss.

- If a pregnant woman is undernourished, obese or has a metabolic disease, this may influence the activity of her child's genes through one of two mechanisms. It may change the epigenetic modifications, and therefore the level of activity, in some of her genes, and the child may inherit these changes directly. Alternatively, it may create a nutritional environment in the womb that causes the level of activity in several of the child's genes to change, as if the fetus' genes expect the child to receive the same balance of fats, carbohydrates and proteins after birth that he/she received before birth.

- The telomeres of your chromosomes get shorter as you age. This may be one reason why your risk for several diseases increases as you get older. Reducing stress and consuming antioxidants and nutrients that insure a good supply of methyl groups may help reduce the rate at which your telomeres shrink.

EPILOGUE AND USEFUL INTERNET RESOURCES

We hope this book has enabled you to better understand how your genetic and non-genetic factors influence your health. We hope you now see that family history is an important tool to help you and your healthcare team better understand your risk for certain diseases and design a health management plan that is best for you based on this information. We also hope you have learned that personalized medicine sees each person's body as an integrated ecosystem, with the different elements of the ecosystem (genetic, dietary, environmental, lifestyle, experience) influencing each other, and mechanisms in place to keep the different aspects of the ecosystem in balance with each other. In addition, the best personalized medicine tests will need to take into account the fact that the degree to which genetic factors and nongenetic factors influence your risk for a specific disease may change over the course of your life. Indeed, there are many challenges ahead, and it will require a lot of time and research to truly bring out the full potential of personalized medicine. It is also true, however, that the new technologies have enabled researchers to gather unprecedented amounts of data, and it is just a matter of time before we know how to use this information to improve health care for everyone.

We also think you can predict the way in which the field of personalized medicine will expand by looking at the evolution of computer technology. Not only will the development of the field of personalized medicine resemble the development of the computer technology field, the developments that have occurred in the computer technology field are an important part of what is enabling the field of personalized medicine to evolve as it is evolving. The advances in computer chip technology have enabled the field of computer technology to advance to where we can hold computers in our hand that are more powerful than computers that used to take up an entire room. Applying computer chip technology to genetic analyses has enabled the development of microarray-based assays that provide researchers with overwhelming amounts of data in a single experiment. In addition, the advances in DNA sequence analysis programs are enabling researchers to make sense out of these massive bodies of information much more quickly than was ever possible. Just as we went from room-sized computers that were slow and limited in their capabilities to palm-sized computers that can run thousands of applications, we will go from single-gene tests that give sometimes vague information about risk for disease and response to treatment to whole-genome sequencing and personalized medicine programs that combine information about your

DNA sequence, clinical data such as blood sugar level, family history, age, sex, diet and job-related environmental exposures to provide startlingly accurate estimates of your risk for diseases, or likely response to a drug.

Personalized medicine will not only allow doctors to treat sick people more safely and effectively, it will also allow people to take a more active role in their own health care. By identifying the diseases for which you have the greatest genetic risk, you can identify the nongenetic factors you must reduce your exposure to in order to reduce your overall chance of developing those diseases. You can also design a plan for regular health screenings and tests that focus on the diseases for which you have the greatest risk. By using your genetic information wisely, you and your doctor can reduce your chances of ever getting sick, as well as design safer and more effective treatments when you do. We hope this book will help you play your part in this process. After all, you are the person who is most responsible for maintaining your own health. We hope we have helped you do so.

POTENTIALLY USEFUL RESOURCES

There are several Internet websites that house resources that can help you further understand the foundational principles underlying personalized medicine and the ways in which this information is applied to improve health care.

The National Human Genome Research Institute, which is a division of the National Institute of Health, maintains a website at which you can find a wide variety of educational materials: http://www.genome.gov/Education/.

The National Library of Medicine maintains a website that includes an extensive listing of websites where you can find educational materials: http://ghr.nlm.nih.gov/Resources/education.

The Genetic Science Learning Center at the University of Utah has tools to help you further understand both the foundational genetic concepts and some of the ways in which genetic information is being applied to health care: http://learn.genetics.utah.edu/.

Another helpful tool is called "DNA From the Beginning", funded by the Josiah Macy, Jr. Foundation and developed by the Dolan DNA Learning Center: http://www.dnaftb.org/. The Dolan DNA Learning Center has additional materials at: http://www.dnalc.org/.

There is also a comprehensive list of resources hosted by the University of Kansas Medical Center Genetics Education Center at: http://www.kumc.edu/gec/.

There are a number of websites at which you can see videos that animate the process whereby a gene makes its protein. Open your favorite web browser and use "transcription" and "translation" as search terms.

The National Institute of General Medical Sciences Pharmacogenomics Research Network provides educational materials for those interested in how genomic information is being used to guide decisions about prescribing drugs: http://www.nigms.nih.gov/Initiatives/PGRN/Education.htm.

The Department of Energy Human Genome Project Information website includes information on basic genetics, gene therapy, genetic testing, pharmacogenomics, and ethical, legal and social issues: http://www.ornl.gov/sci/techresources/Human_Genome/project/about.shtml.

The Centers for Disease Control and Prevention maintain a Public Health Genomics website, with links to several programs and publications, including the weekly email bulletin that reports on news articles and literature that focus on genetic and genomic issues: http://www.cdc.gov/genomics/.

Several websites focus on the ethical, legal and social issues that are associated with personalized medicine, including: http://www.genomicslawreport.com and http://scienceblogs.com/geneticfuture/.

INDEX